NHS
DATA
BOOK

NHS DATA BOOK

JOHN FRY

General Practitioner, Beckenham, Kent

DAVID BROOKS

General Practitioner, Manchester

IAN McCOLL

Professor of Surgery, Guy's Hospital, London

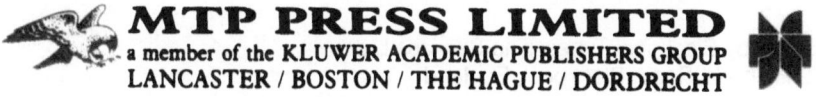

MTP PRESS LIMITED

a member of the KLUWER ACADEMIC PUBLISHERS GROUP

LANCASTER / BOSTON / THE HAGUE / DORDRECHT

Published in the UK and Europe by
MTP Press Limited
Falcon House
Lancaster, England

British Library Cataloguing in Publication Data

Fry, John, *1922*-
    NHS data book.
    1. Great Britain—National Health Service—
    Statistics
    I. Title   II. Brooks, David, *19----*
    III. McColl, Ian
    362.1'0941   RA395.G6

    ISBN-13:978-94-010-8964-7   e-ISBN-13:978-94-009-5590-5

    DOI: 10.1007/978-94-009-5590-5

Published in the USA by
MTP Press
A division of Kluwer Boston Inc
190 Old Derby Street
Hingham, MA 02043, USA

Library of Congress Cataloging in Publication Data
Fry, John, 1922-
    NHS data book.

    Includes index.
    1. Great Britain—Statistics, Medical. 2. Great
    Britain—National Health Service—Statistics.
    3. Great Britain—Population—Statistics. I. Brooks,
    David, M.D. II. McColl, Ian. III. Title. IV. Title:
    N.H.S. data book. [DNLM: 1. State medicine—Great
    Britain. W 275 FA1 F9n]
    RA407.5.G7F78 1984   362.1'0941   84-3895

Typeset by Blackpool Typesetting Services Ltd.,
132 Highfield Road, Blackpool, England

CONTENTS

	Preface	vii
Chapter 1	Population	1
Chapter 2	Socioeconomic factors	13
Chapter 3	Mortality and morbidity in a district	35
Chapter 4	Social pathologies	49
Chapter 5	Inequalities in health correlates of social class	73
Chapter 6	Structure and roles of NHS	87
Chapter 7	Facilities and resources	91
Chapter 8	Personnel in NHS	105
Chapter 9	Education, training and careers	121
Chapter 10	Utilization of resources and content of work	129
Chapter 11	Prescribing	155
Chapter 12	Psychiatry	163
Chapter 13	Maternity services	179
Chapter 14	Eyes and teeth	185
Chapter 15	School medical service	193
Chapter 16	Quality and outcomes	197
Chapter 17	Complaints	249
Chapter 18	Costs	259
	Index	269

PREFACE

Administering the National Health Service (NHS) is asking to navigate without reliable and sufficient information. It is amazing how a national service costing more than £15,000M (1984) and employing more than 1 million has existed since 1948. It is likely that with better appropriate data there could be economies and great efficiency and effectiveness.

Paradoxically there is much data on the NHS, published and unpublished, that has remained unexploited and unused.

In this book we have taken up the challenges of showing the availability of data and its presentation so that clinicians, administrators, committee members and politicians can better understand the state and needs of the NHS.

Why this book? Because it is not possible to make decisions without facts. There is too much data around that is unrelated to the needs of clinicians, administrators, committee members and politicians. It can be brought together to provide bases for decisions and, more important, to show the gaps that exist and the need for more information.

What does it contain? It includes social and demographic data, NHS facts and figures, manpower data on the use of the NHS and some examples of how quality can be assessed and promoted.

Where does the information come from? No extra research was carried out to collect new data. Our main sources were the excellent, but neglected, publications from government sources, and particularly *Health and Personal Social Services Statistics, England* and *Social Trends* published annually by Her Majesty's Stationery Office. The *Compendia of Health Statistics* published by the Office of Health Economics, London, was invaluable. Answers to Parliamentary Questions in *Hansard* were revealing. Also we used some other sources that were known to us.

How? We have attempted to present information factually and pictorially with minimum of text, not to provide all the answers, but to suggest trends and patterns for readers to follow up.

We hope that we have excited our readers to pause, reflect and to take actions that should lead to an even better NHS.

JOHN FRY,
Beckenham, 1984

Acknowledgements

Our sincere thanks are due to the Controller of Her Majesty's Stationery Office to reproduce material from its publications; to George Teeling-Smith for allowing us to reproduce from OHE *Compendia*; and to Sir Henry Yellowlees and his colleagues at the Department of Health and Social Services for unpublished data.

CHAPTER 1

POPULATION

UK POPULATION

Since 1901 the population of the UK has grown at a mean rate of 2.2 million every 10 years but with a marked reduction in rate of increase in the last decade 1971–1981. The estimates for the next 20 years also are for smaller increases (see Table 1).

Table 1   UK population 1901–2001

	Population (millions)	Changes every 10 years (millions)
1901	38.2	
1911	42.1	+3.9
1921	44.0	+1.9
1931	46.0	+2.0
1941	—	
1951	50.3	+3.7
1961	52.8	+2.5
1971	55.6	+2.8
1981	55.9	+0.3
1991 (Estimate)	57.2	+1.3
2001 (Estimate)	58.0	+0.8
1901–2001	+19.8	+1.98 every 10 years

Source: Social Trends, 1982, Table 1.2

UK Population 1980

In 1980 the age–sex distribution shows how the ups and downs in births influence the structure. Always more boys are born than girls. As they grow, more men than women die earlier and from the age of 50 women outnumber men (Figure 2).

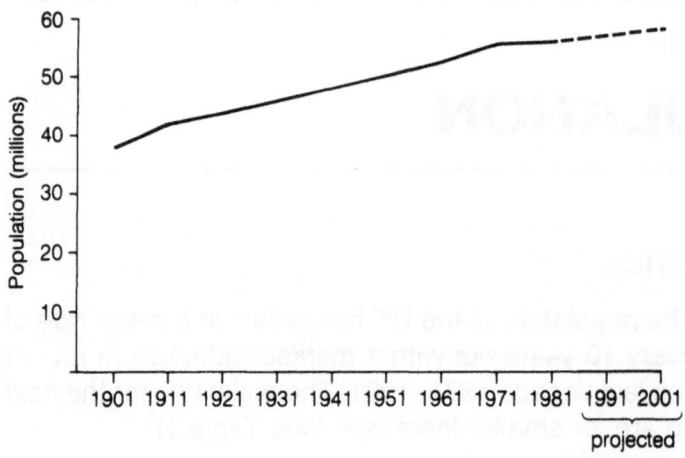

*Figure 1   UK Population 1901–2001 (*Social Trends, *1982, Table 1.2)*

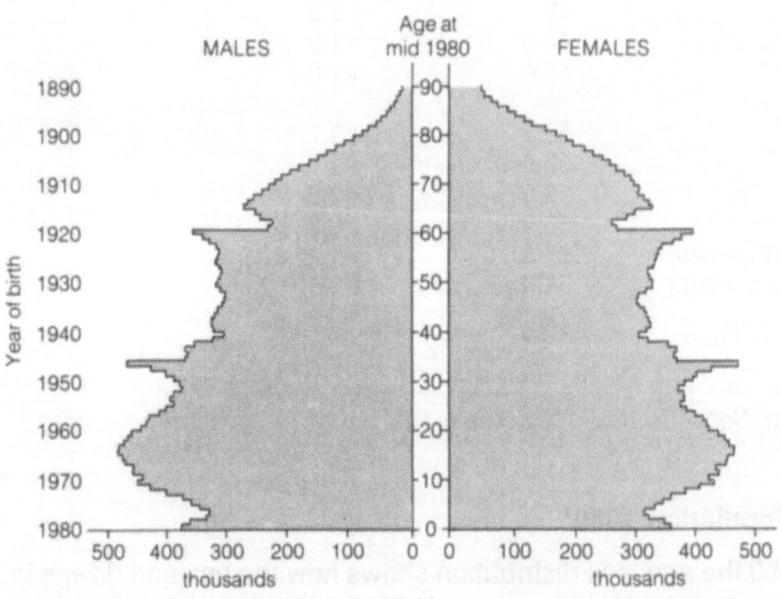

*Figure 2   UK Population by age and sex, 1980 (*Social Trends, *1982, Chart 1.1)*

Figures 3–5 illustrate the trends in numbers of children, elderly and all dependents from 1961 to 2001. Figure 3 shows the decline in numbers of children in the 1980s as a result of the fall in birth rate in the 1970s. Figure 4 shows that over 17 per cent of the population are now over 65 years of age, compared with 15 per cent in 1961. Projections suggest that numbers of very old (75–84) and very very old (85+) will increase; those aged 65–74 will decrease. Figure 5 shows that the 'dependent' population, of children and retired elderly, as a proportion of those of working age, is about two-thirds. This means that for every 20 persons of working age there are 13 dependents (*Social Trends*, 1982).

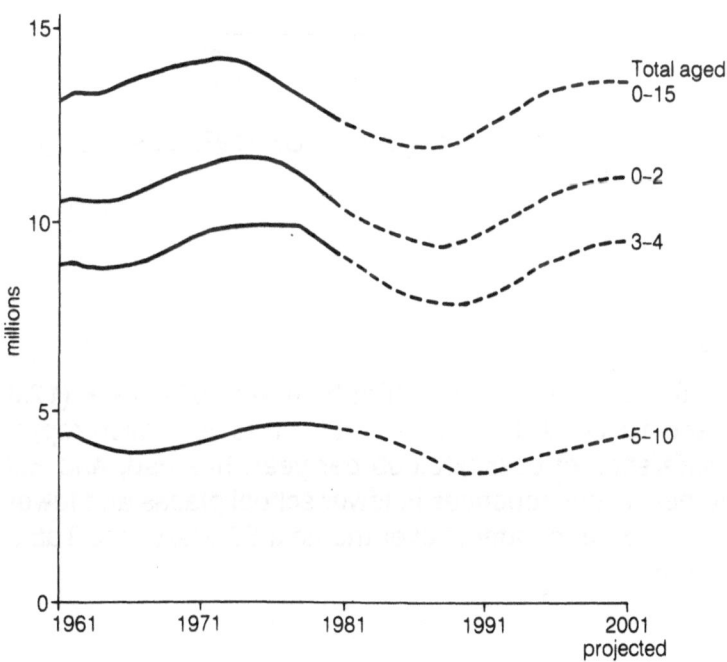

Figure 3   Children: by age group – UK (1979-based projections)

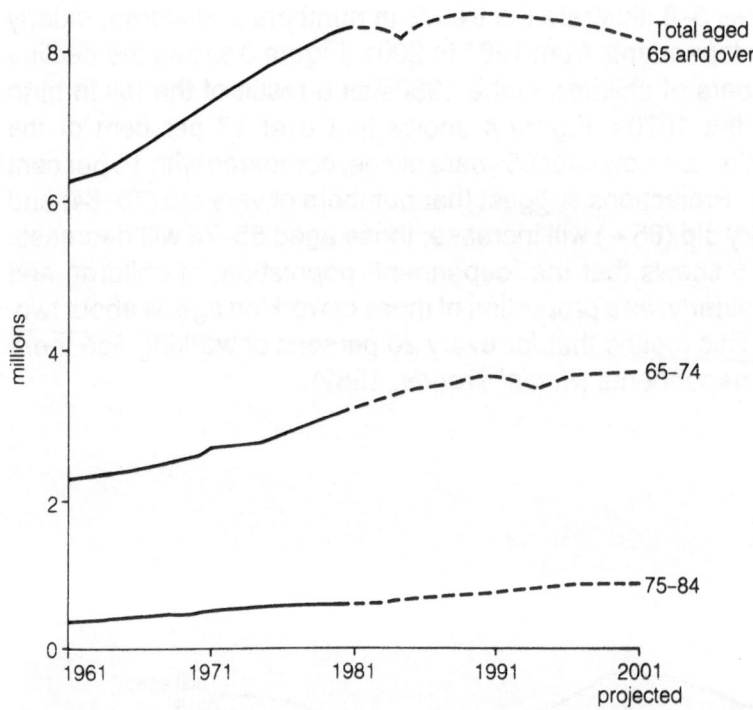

Figure 4   Elderly people: by age group – UK (1979-based projections)

Live births

The birth rate fell by almost one-third between 1961–1976 (17.8 per 1000) and 1976–1981 (11.9 per 1000). This fall, which represented a difference of over 300,000 per year, has had, and will continue to have, consequences in fewer school places and fewer workers to support dependents over the next 50 years (see Table 2 and Figure 6).

Deaths

Death rates (per 1000 of population) remain relatively constant (Figure 7) – mean annual rate of 11.8 per 1000 or 30 per GP.

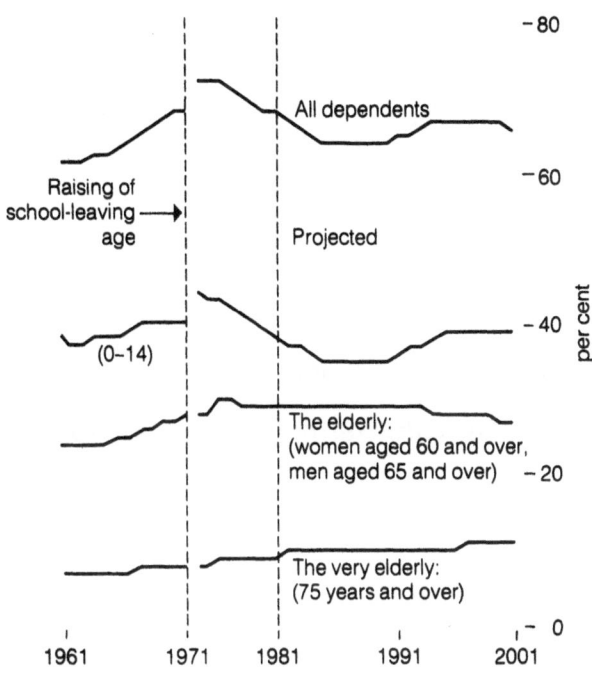

Figure 5   The dependent population (UK) as a percentage of the
population of working age (1979-based projections)

Table 2   Annual birth rates (UK) 1951–1981

	Annual live births		
Year	Per 1000 of population	Per GP with 2500 patients	Per District General Hospital serving 250,000 persons (to nearest 100)
1951	15.7	39	3900
1956	16.0	40	4000
1961	17.8	45	4500
1966	17.8	45	4500
1971	16.1	40	4000
1976	11.9	30	3000
1981	13.4	32	3200

Source: *Social Trends*, 1982, Table 1.12

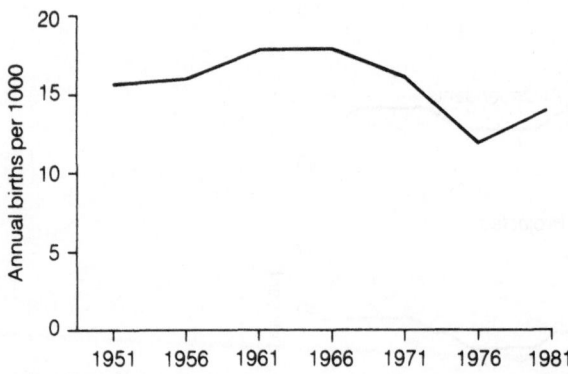

*Figure 6 Annual birth rates (UK) 1951–1981 (*Social Trends, *1982, Table 1.12)*

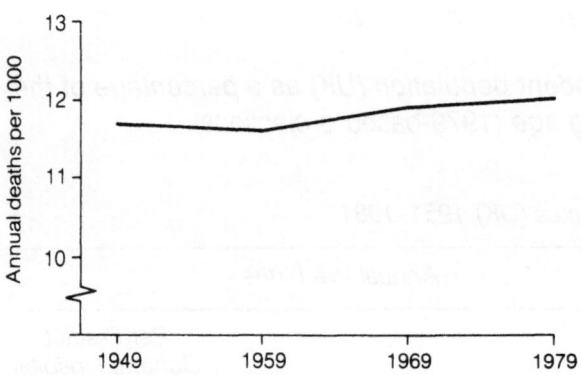

*Figure 7 Annual death rates (UK) 1949–1979 (*Health and Personal Social Services Statistics for England, *1982, Table 1.1)*

CAUSES OF DEATH

In 1980 there were 544,000 deaths in England. The top seven causes of death are shown in Table 3 and Figure 8. They accounted for two-thirds of all deaths. The rates related to a GP and a DGH show the numbers that may be expected in a year.

6   POPULATION

Table 3   Causes of deaths in England, 1980

Causes of death	Numbers for England in 1980 (to nearest 1000)	Per GP with 2500 patients	Per District General Hospital serving 250,000 persons (to nearest 100)
Ischaemic heart disease	145,000	5	500
Cerebrovascular diseases	67,000	3	300
Cancers	60,000	3	300
Pneumonia	50,000	2	200
Bronchitis	18,000	1	100
Accidents	15,000	1 every 2 years	50
Suicide	4000	1 every 6 years	15
Total	544,000	20	2000

Source: *Health and Personal Social Services Statistics for England*, 1982, Table 1.4

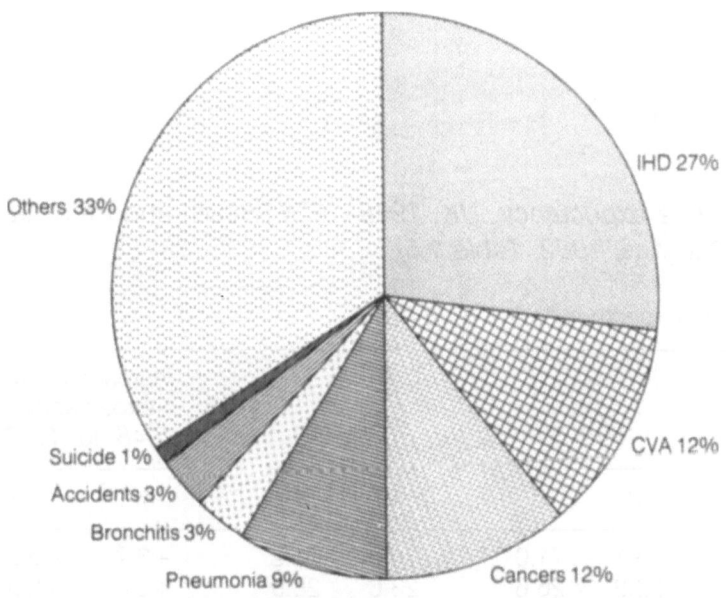

Figure 8   Causes of death in England, 1980 (Health and Personal Social Services Statistics for England, 1982, Table 1.4)

Life expectancy

Women have always lived longer than men and there have always been more male babies born than female. At the other end of life (over 75 years) there are twice as many women as men in the UK. Note (Figure 9 and Table 4) that at all ages the life expectancy over the 30 years 1948–1978 increased in both sexes, but by 5.2 years in females and 3.7 years in males. Note also that at 50 years the increase in life expectancy in males has been only 0.8 years and for females 2.3 years, and, at 65, 0.3 in males and 2.0 years in females.

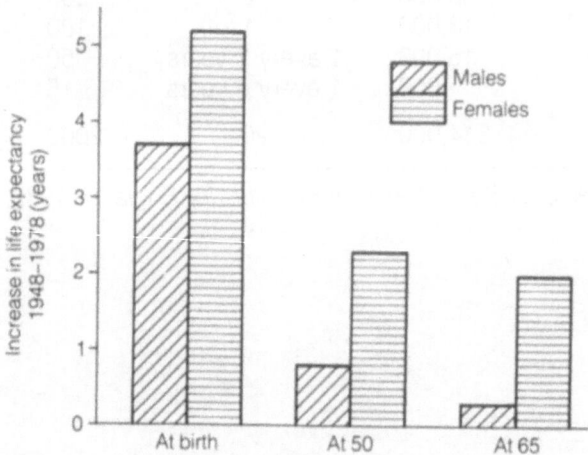

*Figure 9   Life expectancy, UK, 1948–1978 (*Health and Personal Services Statistics, *1982, Table 1.5)*

Table 4   Life expectancy (UK) 1948–1978

	1948–50		1976–78		Increased life expectancy 1948 to 1978	
	M	F	M	F	M	F
At birth	66.3	71.0	70.0	76.2	+3.7	+5.2
At 50	22.8	26.6	23.6	28.9	+0.8	+2.3
At 65	12.2	14.6	12.5	16.6	+0.3	+2.0

Source: *Health and Personal Services Statistics*, 1982, Table 1.5

Migration

From 1964 to 1980 there was a net excess of emigration over immigration in the UK of 600,000 (Figure 10 and Table 5).

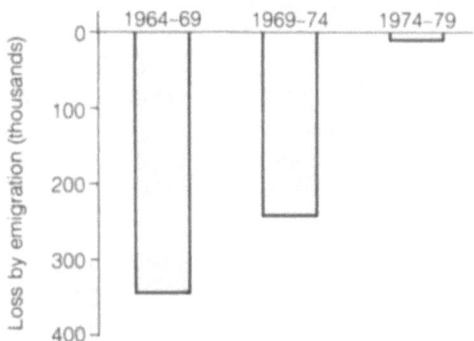

Figure 10 Migration to and from the UK, 1964–1980 (Social Trends, *1982, Table 1.16)*

Table 5   Migration to and from the UK, 1964–1980

	Numbers (000's)		
Years	Immigration (in)	Emigration (out)	Net loss
1964–1969	1132	1476	−344
1969–1974	1055	1297	−242
1974–1979	926	936	−10
1979–1980	205	209	−4
Total numbers 1964–1980	3,318,000	3,918,000	−600,000

Source: *Social Trends*, 1982, Table 1.16

WORLD POPULATION

In 1980 the population of the world was estimated by the United Nations to be 4500 million. The population of selected countries in 7 grades is shown in Table 6. Note that the Low Countries (Netherlands and Belgium) were the most densely populated, and Canada and Australia the least densely populated.

Table 6   World populations and density of population, 1980

	Country	Population (millions)	Density of population per km²
>300 million	China	957	100
	India	664	202
100–300 million	USSR	267	12
	USA	228	24
	Brazil	123	14
	Japan	117	312
50–100 million	West Germany	62	247
	Italy	57	189
	UK	56	229
	France	54	98
20–50 million	Turkey	45	58
	Spain	37	58
	Canada	24	2
10–20 million	Australia	15	2
	Netherlands	14	415
5–10 million	Portugal	9.9	108
	Greece	9.6	73
	Sweden	8.3	18
	Belgium	5.1	319
<5 million	Eire	3.4	49
	New Zealand	3.1	12
	Others	1241	—
Total world population		4500	

Source: World Health Organization

COMMENT

- The *population* of the UK is at minimum growth and is becoming older.
- *Birth rates* have fallen, but have shown a marginal increase in past 3 years.
- *Life expectancy* is increasing and is now 70 years for males and 76 years for females.
- There are *more males than females* in the under-50s but more females than males in the over-50s. There are twice as many females than males in the over-75s.
- For every 20 *workers* there are now 13 *dependents*, children and elderly, plus another 2 unemployed.
- *Emigration* has always been greater than *immigration*, now there is little of either.
- We have to plan for a no-growth *ageing society* with workers supporting almost as many dependents.

CHAPTER 2

SOCIOECONOMIC FACTORS

INCOME: BENEFIT AND TAXES

Income

We are becoming wealthier with more assets. Total household disposable income (before tax) increased by 24 per cent in real terms allowing for inflation between 1971 and 1981. Real household disposable income per head went up by a similar percentage (21 per cent – see Figure 1).

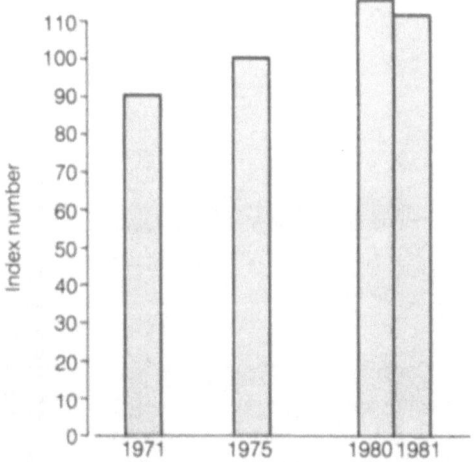

Figure 1   Real household disposable income per head (Social Trends, *1983, Table 5.1)*

Gross weekly earnings

Top earnings for male manual workers in 1981 were in mining, gas, electrical and water supply industries. Earnings were lowest in agriculture, forestry and fishing industries. These top earners

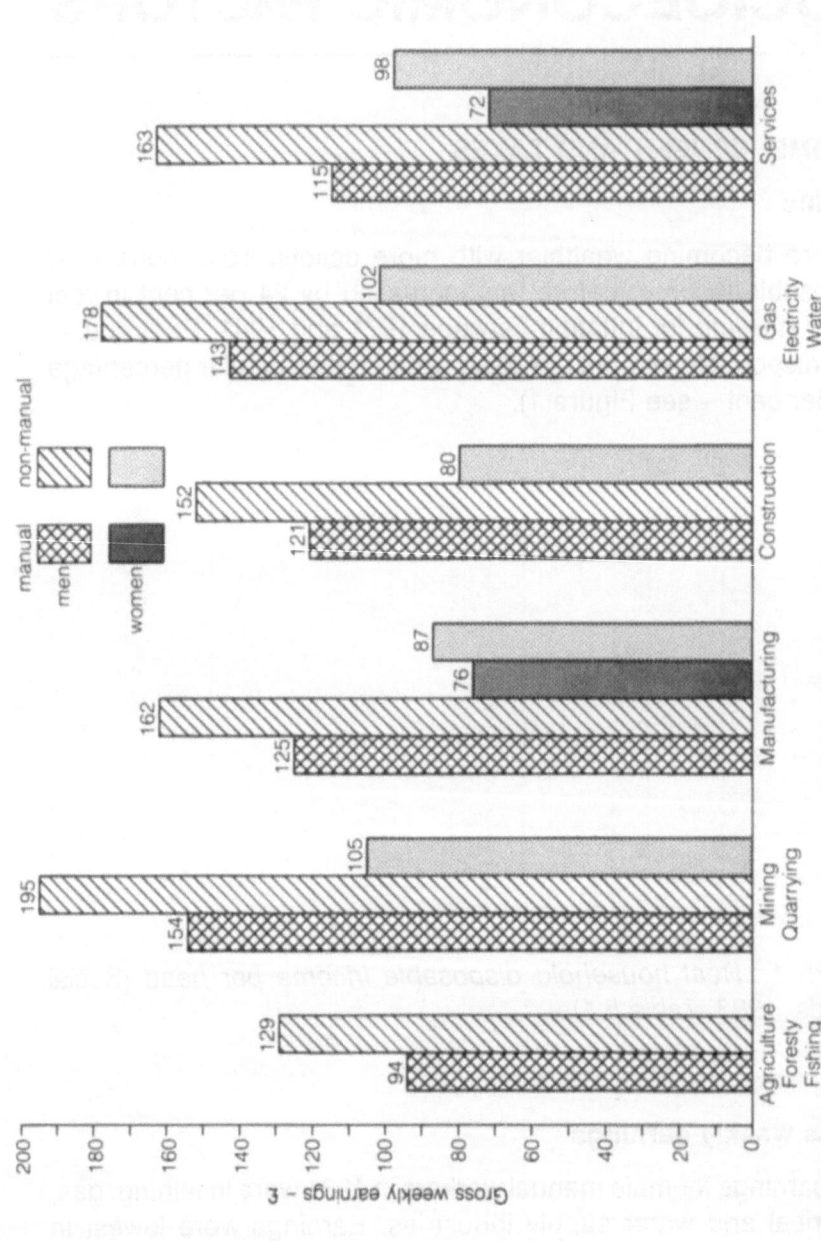

Figure 2 *Weekly earnings for men and women working full-time in different industries (April 1981)*
(Social Trends, 1983, Tables 5.3 and 5.4)

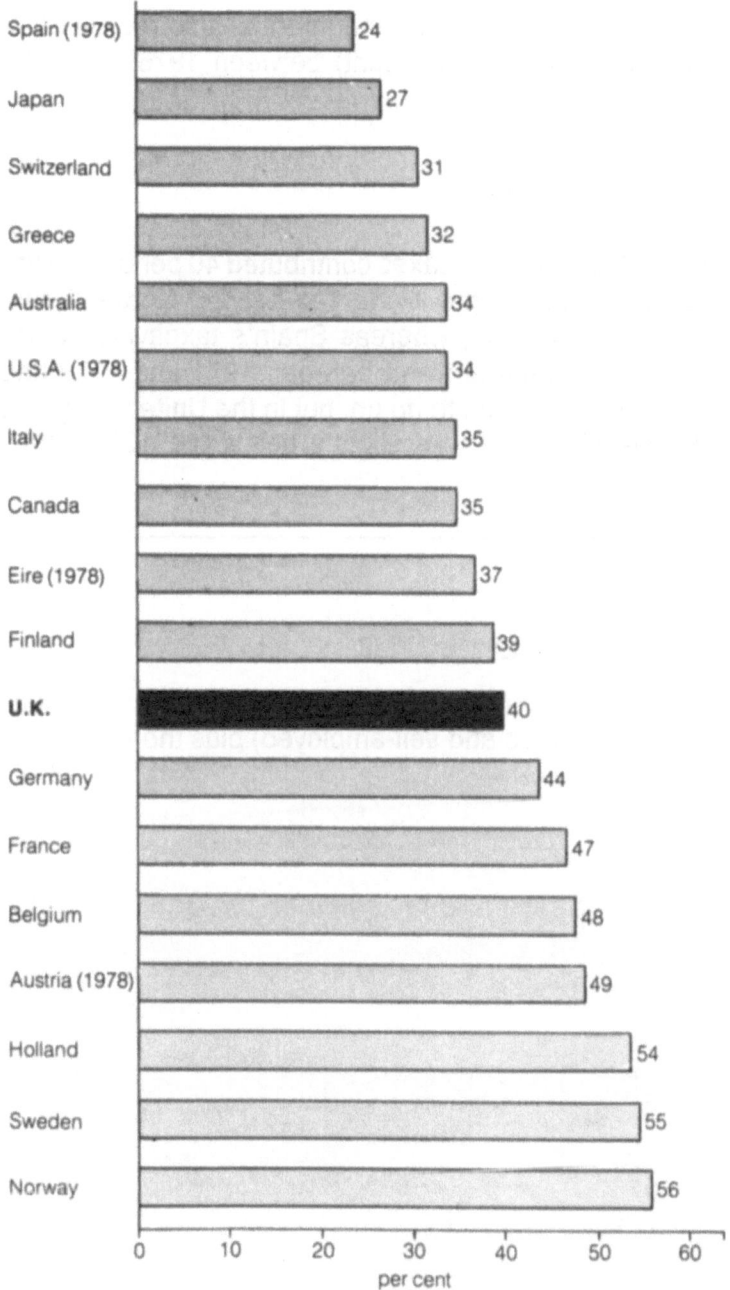

Figure 3   Taxes as a proportion of Gross National Product. World rates in 1979 (Social Trends, *1983, Table 5.9)*

(together with insurance, banking and finance) also received the highest increases (over 100 per cent) between 1976 and 1981 (Figure 2).

Taxes

In 1979 in the United Kingdom taxes contributed 40 per cent to the Gross National Product. In the World Tax League Norway's tax-payers were hit the hardest, whereas Spain's taxpayers contri-buted the least. The general trend between 1971 and 1979 has been for the levels of taxation to go up, but in the United Kingdom and Canada the 1979 rate was slightly below the 1971 figure (Figure 3).

EMPLOYMENT AND UNEMPLOYMENT

The *working population* consists of the employed labour force (full-time, part-time, HM forces and self-employed) plus the registered

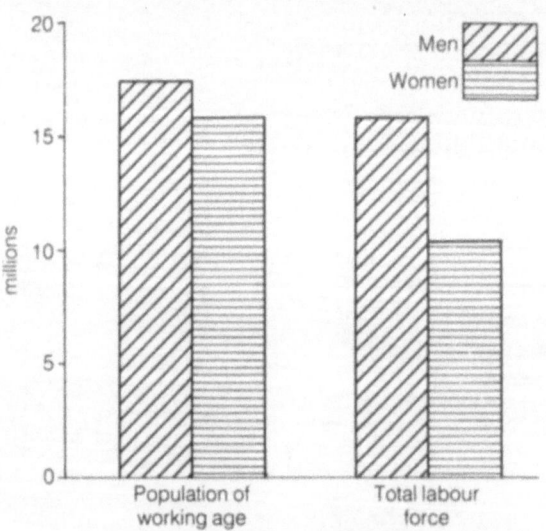

*Figure 4   Labour force and population of working age in the UK in 1979 (*Social Trends, *1983, Table 4.1)*

unemployed. The *total labour force* includes the unregistered unemployed plus the economically inactive (e.g. students) (Figure 4). Thus 93 per cent of males of working age are potential workers and 66 per cent of females.

Employment by industry

Most people are employed in the service industries, which have twice as many employees as the manufacturing industries (Figure 5).

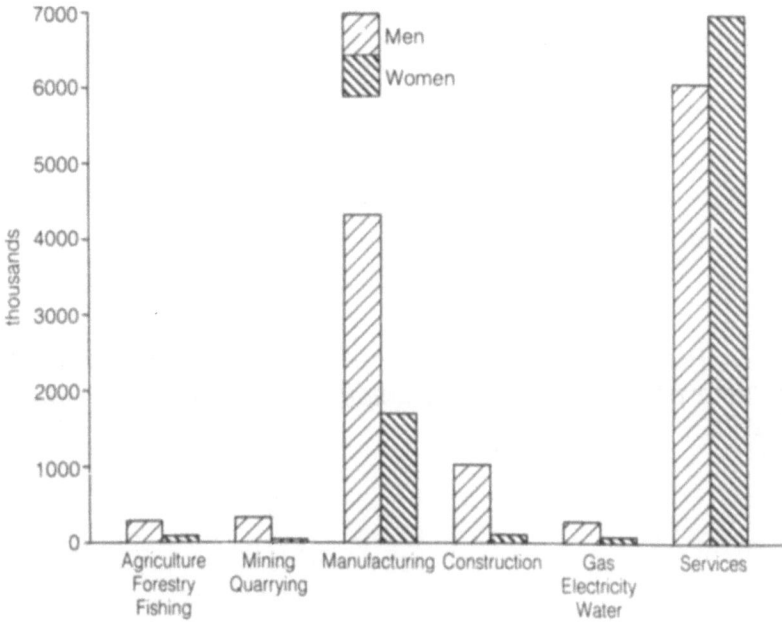

Figure 5   The distribution of the employed working population in 1981 in the United Kingdom (Social Trends, *1983, Table 4.5*)

People in employment by sector

In 1981 nearly one-third of the 23 million people in employment were in the public sector and two-thirds were in the private sector

(Figure 6). The public proportion increased over 20 years (1961–1981).

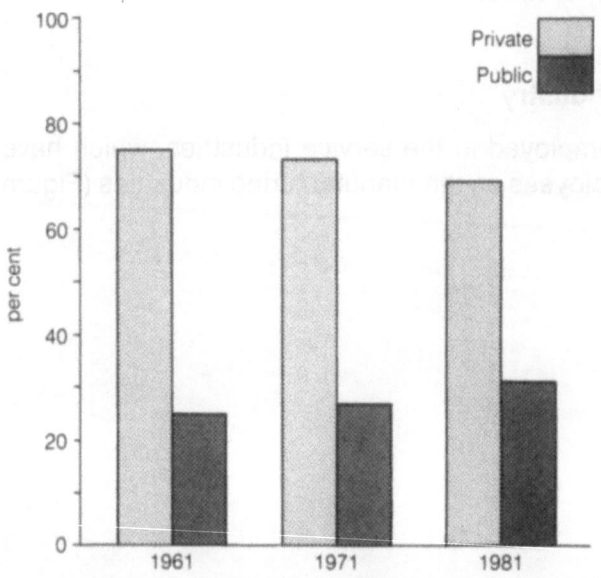

*Figure 6   People in employment by sector United Kingdom 1961 –1981 as a percentage of those employed (*Social Trends, *1983, Table 4.7)*

The unemployed

The unemployed rate was 1.5 per cent in 1961. It has increased by a factor of more than eight over 21 years (1961–1982) (Figure 7).

Unemployment among men and women

The rate is higher in men (Figure 8). Total unemployment rate is 12.5 per cent.

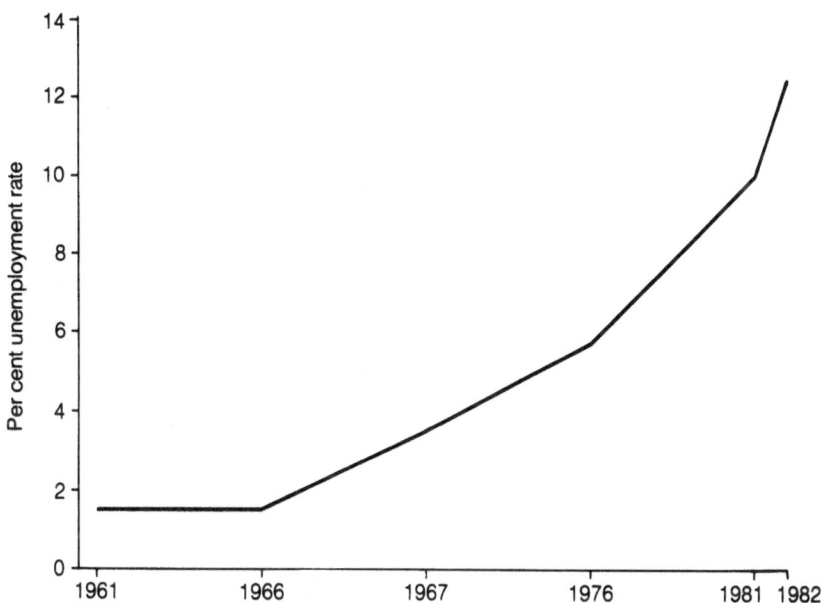

Figure 7   The rise in unemployment: registered unemployed as a percentage of total labour force (Social Trends, 1983, Table 4.13)

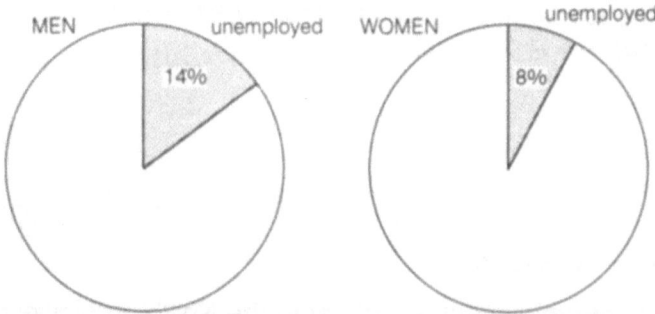

Figure 8   Unemployment rates by sex in 1982 (Social Trends, 1983, Table 4.13)

Unemployment by country

Unemployment is not evenly spread throughout the United Kingdom, being highest in Northern Ireland and lowest in England in 1981 (Figure 9).

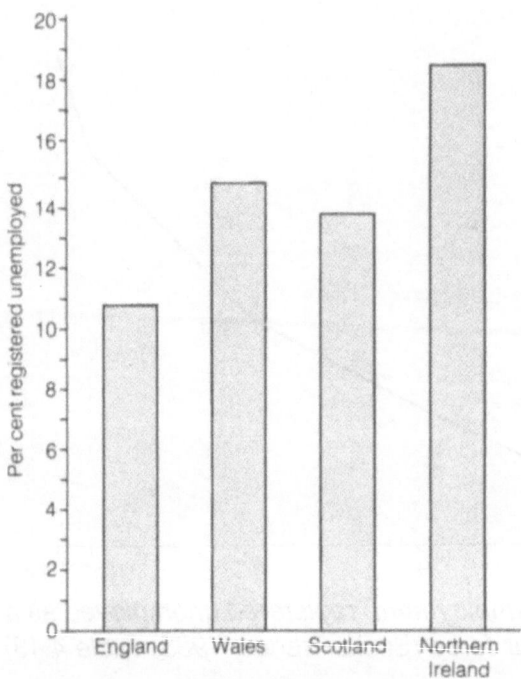

*Figure 9 Unemployment rates by region in 1981 (*Social Trends, *1983, Table 4.14)*

Unemployment in England

Within England unemployment is highest in the North and lowest in the South East (Figure 10).

International comparisons

Great Britain has the highest rate for unemployment in any of the countries shown. The rate has risen particularly steeply since 1980 (Figure 11). Japan is the only country that has escaped unemployment in developed countries.

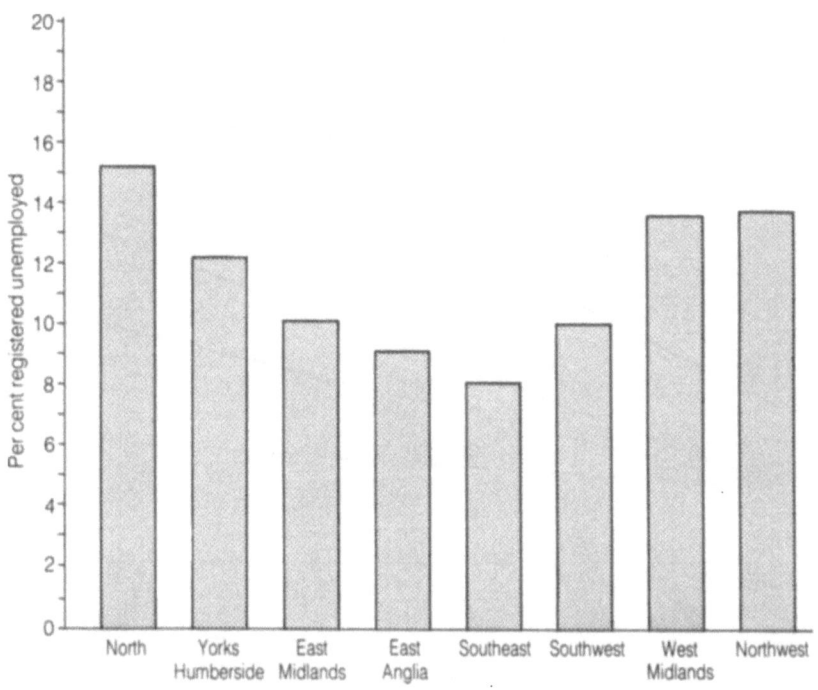

Figure 10   Unemployment in England by standard region in 1981
(Social Trends, *1983, Table 4.14)*

Education and employment

Those with qualifications are more likely to be employed and stay employed (Figure 12).

Time spent at work

Basic hours of full-time employees and overtime have both decreased during the last decade, particularly for non-manual workers, whereas holiday entitlement has increased (Figure 13).

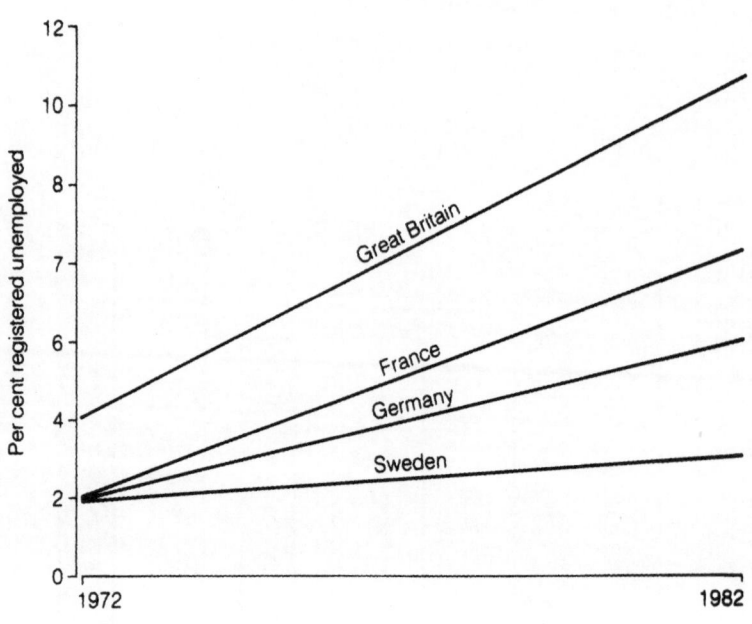

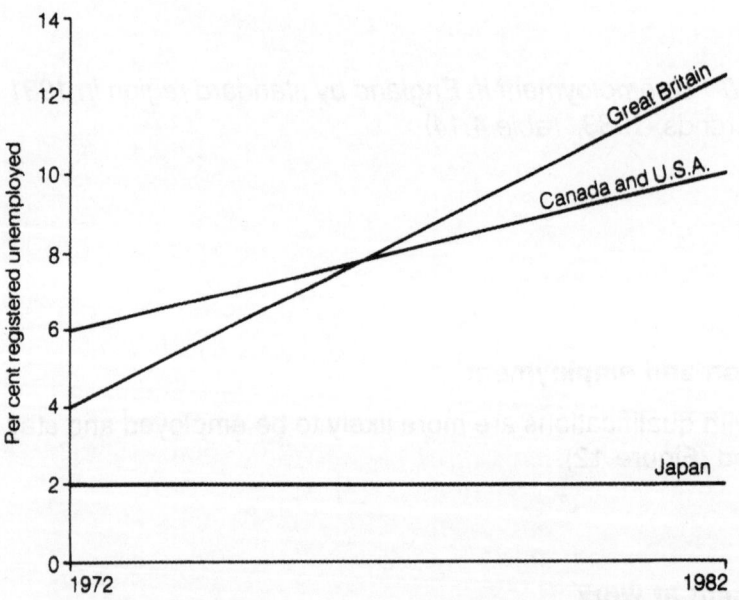

Figure 11 (a) Unemployment in Europe 1972–1982; (b) unem-ployment in Great Britain, Canada and the USA, and Japan (Social Trends, *1983, Chart 4.19)*

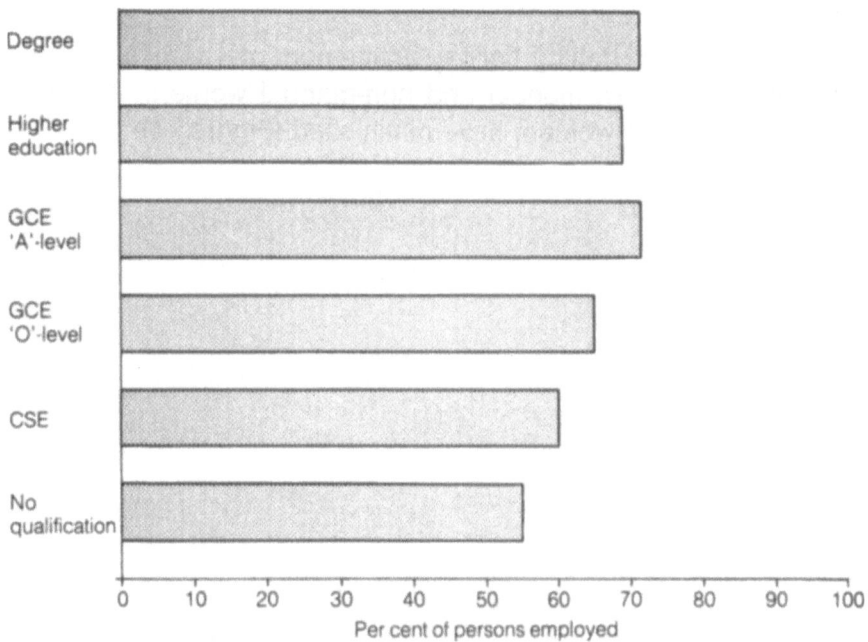

*Figure 12   Percentages employed and educational achievements in women 1980–1981 (*Social Trends, *1983, Chart 4.8)*

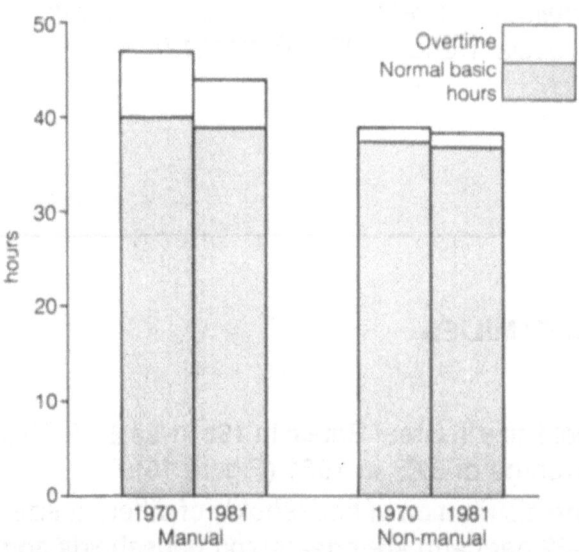

*Figure 13   Average weekly hours worked for full-time male employees in Great Britain (*Social Trends, *1983, Chart 4.9)*

Holidays

More people are getting holiday entitlement of 4 weeks or more. The gaps between manual and non-manual workers, and non-manual men and women, have diminished (Figure 14).

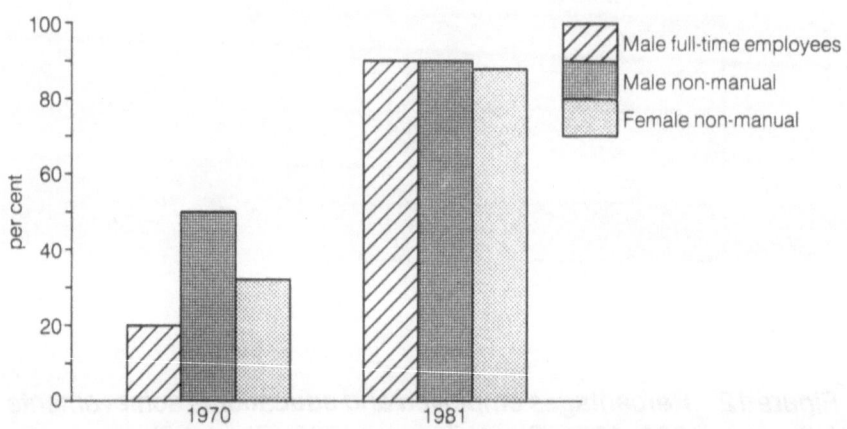

*Figure 14   Annual holiday entitlement 1970–1981 of 4 weeks or more, Great Britain (*Social Trends, *1983, Table 4.12)*

HOUSEHOLDS AND FAMILIES

Household size

The average household size in Great Britain in 1981 was 2.71. This was a fall from an average of 3.09 in 1961 (Figure 15).

Figure 16 shows the distribution of households of different size. Almost one-quarter (22 per cent) are one-person households and more than one-half are one- and two-person households. Large households of six or more are few (4 per cent).

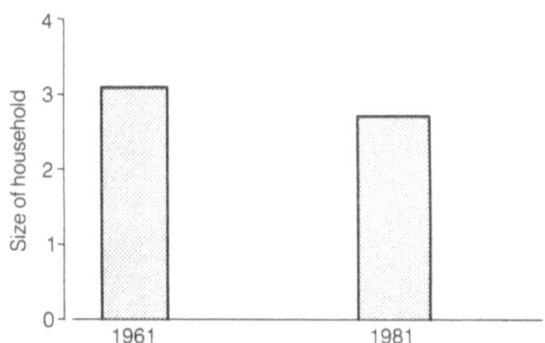

*Figure 15 Households – average persons per household 1961
and 1981 (*Social Trends, *1983, Table 2.3)*

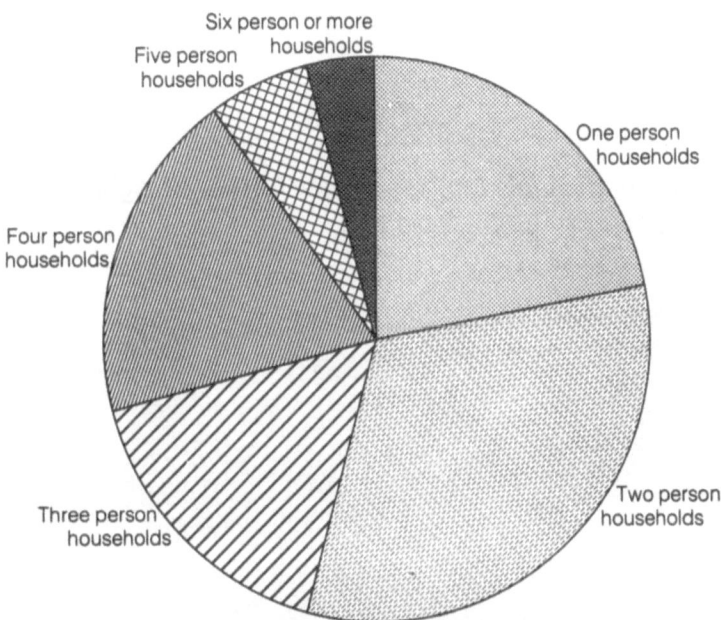

*Figure 16 Households – percentages of persons per household
(1981) (*Social Trends, *1983, Table 2.3)*

Married households

Of married couples more than one-half have no children living with
them (Figure 17).

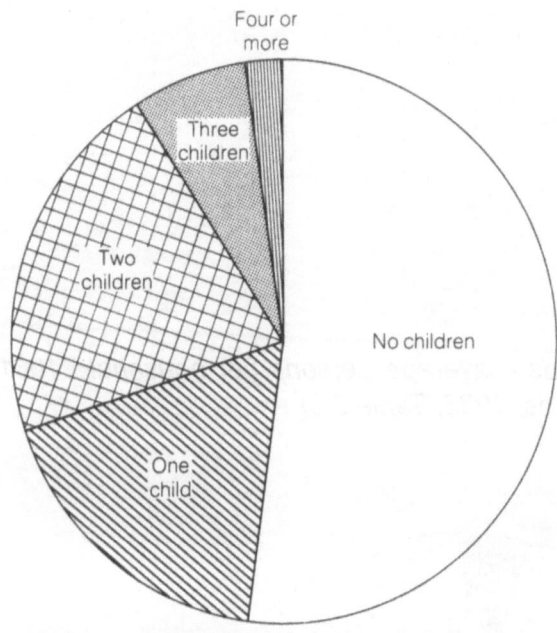

Figure 17 Married couple families by size in 1981 all ages, Great Britain (Social Trends, *1983, Table 2.6*)

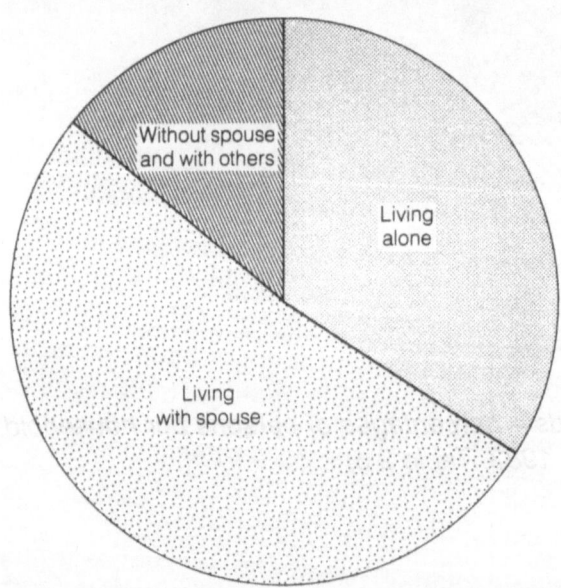

Figure 18 People over 65 and where they lived in 1980–1981, Great Britain (Social Trends, *1983, Table 2.4*)

The elderly

About one-third of elderly people in the community live alone. (Figure 18). This proportion is much higher for women; one-half of women over 75 live alone.

HOUSING, TENURE AND STANDARDS OWNERSHIP

In 1981 more persons owned their homes than in 1961 (Figure 19).

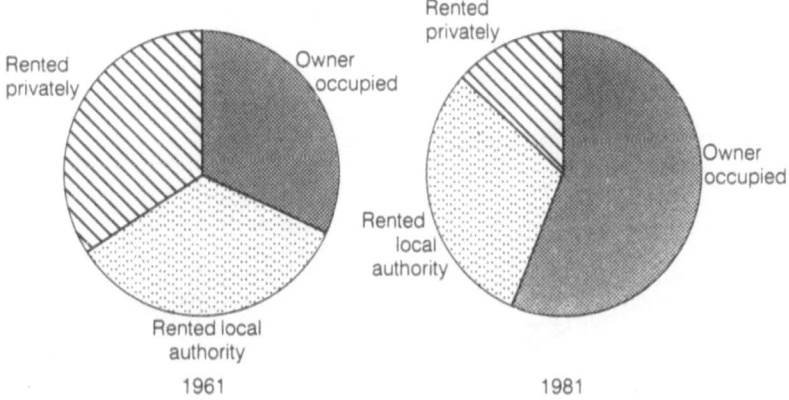

Figure 19   House ownership in Great Britain, 1961 and 1981 (Social Trends, *1983, Table 8.6)*

Standards

Housing standards improved between 1971 and 1981 (Figure 20), but standards still varied by the age of the property (Figure 21).

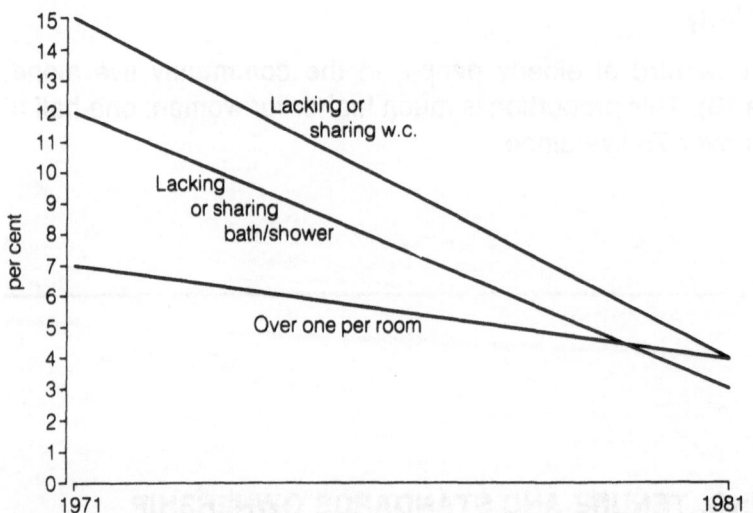

Figure 20 Households lacking basic amenities 1971–1981, Great Britain (Social Trends, 1983, Table 8.9)

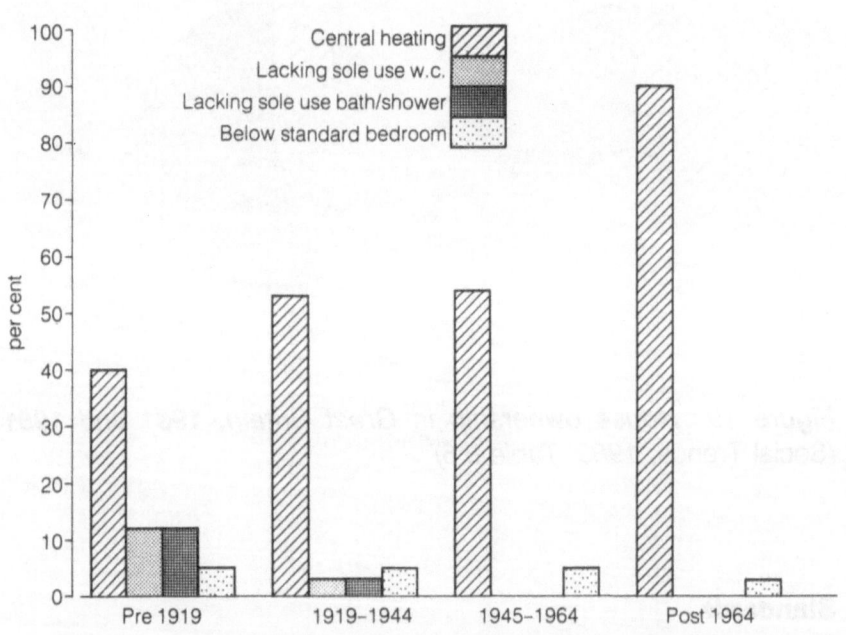

Figure 21 Households by housing standards and age of building, Great Britain, 1981 (Social Trends, 1983, Table 8.11)

Amenities

The percentage of households with regular use of a car, and the percentage of households with a telephone, both increased over the last two decades (Figures 22 and 23).

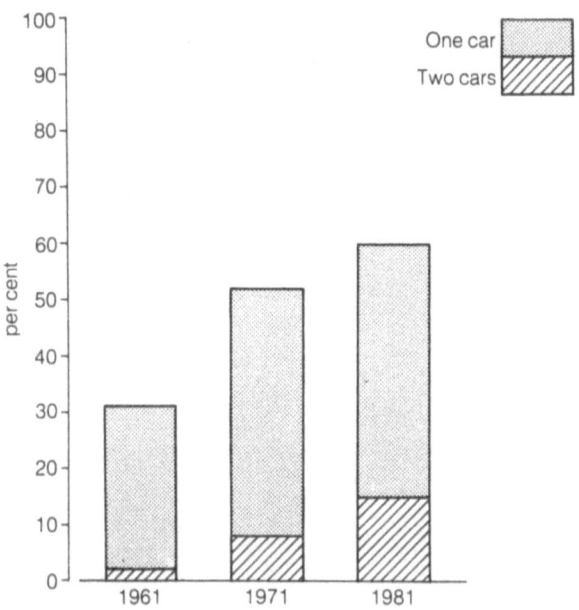

Figure 22   Households with regular use of a car, Great Britain (Social Trends, *1983, Table 6.12*)

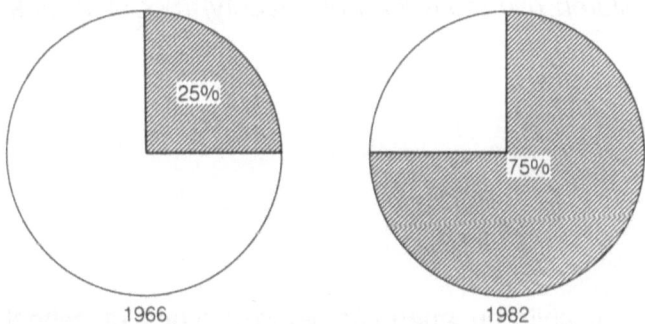

Figure 23   Households with a telephone, United Kingdom (Social Trends, *1983, Table 6.12*)

EDUCATION

The under-fives

Nearly half the under-fives are receiving day care of some sort.
(Figure 24).

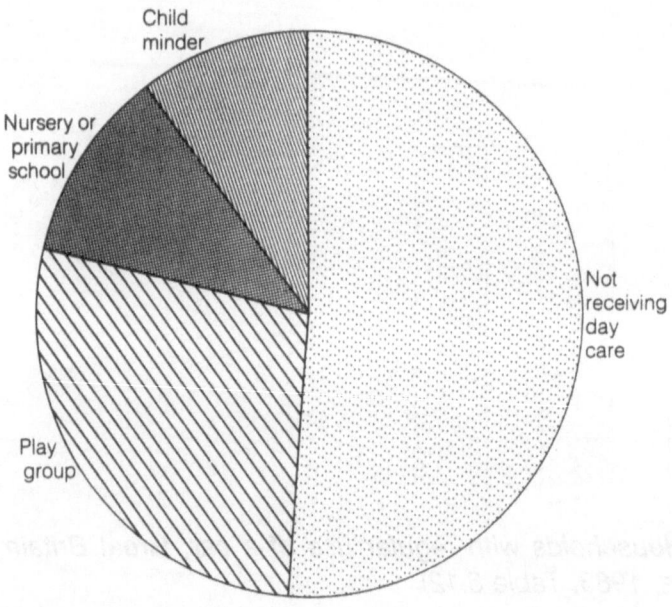

*Figure 24   Type of care facility for the under-fives in 1979, Great
Britain (some children use more than one facility) (Social Trends,
1983, Table 3.3)*

School pupils

The proportions of children attending various types of school
(Figure 25) show that only 6 per cent of children were at private fee-
paying independent schools, and that 94 per cent of schoolchildren
receive a state education.

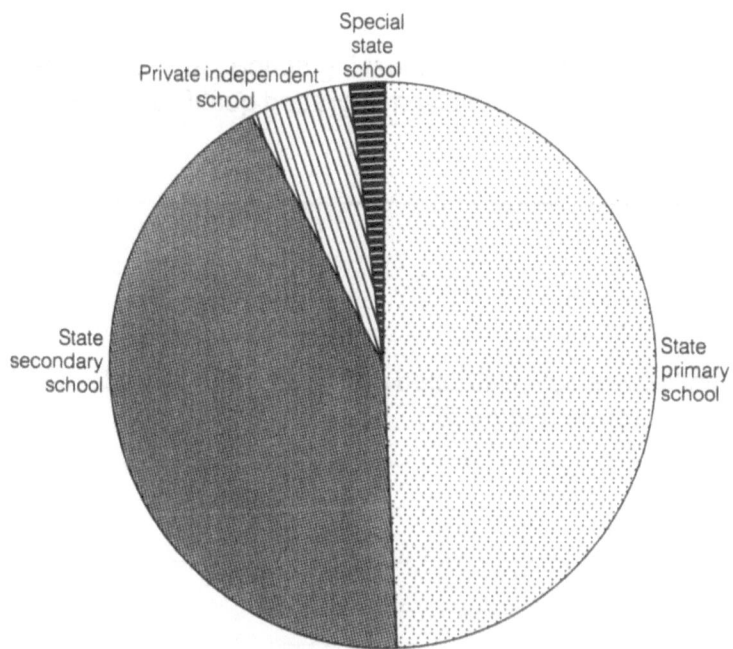

Figure 25   School pupils by type of school, United Kingdom, 1981 (Social Trends, *1983, Table 3.4)*

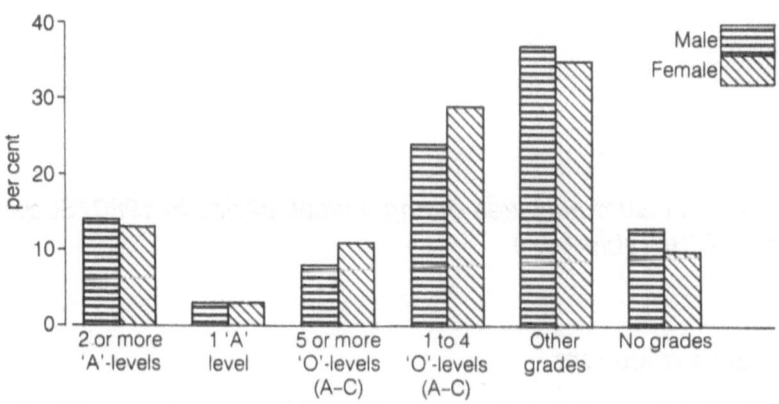

Figure 26   Highest qualification of school-leavers, 1980–1981, England (Social Trends, *1983, Chart 3.8)*

School-leavers

Eighty-seven per cent of all boys leaving school, and 90 per cent of all girls, have achieved some sort of graded qualification (Figure 26).

LEISURE

Most popular leisure activities listed during a 4-week period in 1980 showed a wide range (Figure 27).

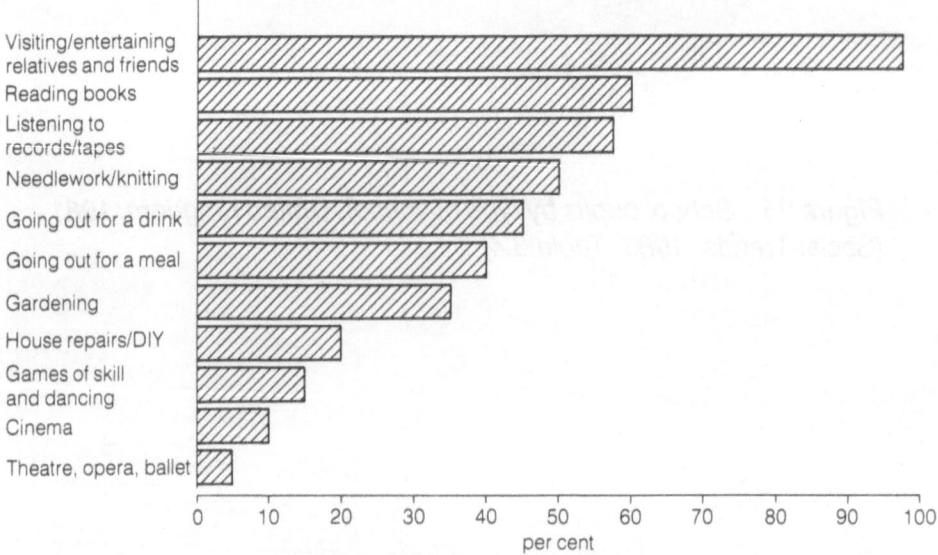

*Figure 27 Leisure activities during 4-week period in 1980 (*Social Trends, *1983, Table 10.1)*

National newspapers

The British are great newspaper readers; 70 per cent read at least one paper daily. The average daily circulation for the various papers is shown in Figure 28.

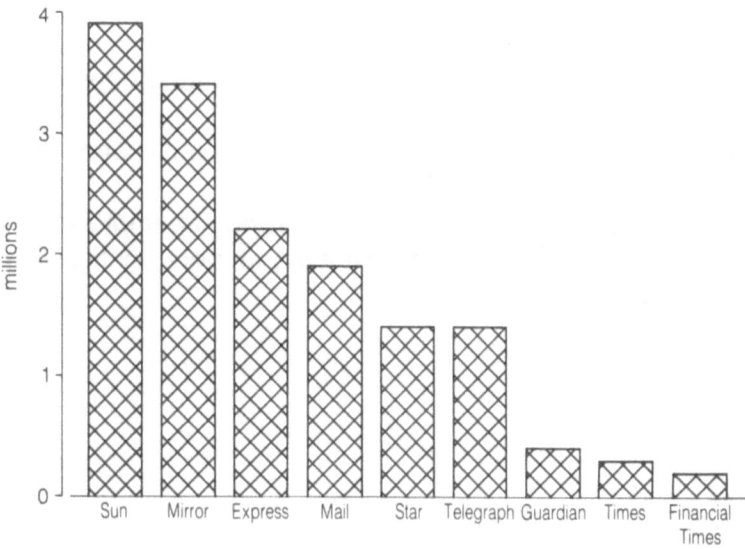

Figure 28 Average daily circulation of British newpapers, 1981
(Social Trends, *1983, Table 10.6)*

COMMENT

- We are wealthier than ever before. In real terms our *wealth* increased by 21 per cent from 1971 to 1981.
- The UK is in the middle of the *tax league*. Taxes are 40 per cent of our GNP. In Norway taxes are 56 per cent and in Spain 24 per cent.
- There are twice as many *employed* in service industries as in manufacturing.
- Two-thirds of *workers* are in the private sector and one-third in the public sector.
- *Unemployment* in UK has increased 10-fold since 1961 and now is the highest of all developed countries.
- *Hours of work* have decreased since 1970 – by 4 hours in manual work (44 hours per week) and by ½ hour in non-manual work (38.5 hours per week).
- Almost all workers have more than 4 weeks *holidays* annually.
- *Standards of housing* have improved, and in 1981 56 per cent were owner-occupiers.

- Forty-five per cent of *families* have a car and 75 per cent a telephone.
- Only 6 per cent of *schoolchildren* attend private independent schools.
- Ninety per cent of *school-leavers* have some qualification – 17 per cent one or more at 'A' level standard.
- In spite of economic difficulties and increasing unemployment, data suggest that we are more *affluent* and more comfortable than ever before.

CHAPTER 3

MORTALITY AND MORBIDITY IN A DISTRICT

A DISTRICT

In an NHS district (Figure 1) there will be over 120 general practitioners and 60 consultants providing medical care for 250,000
persons.

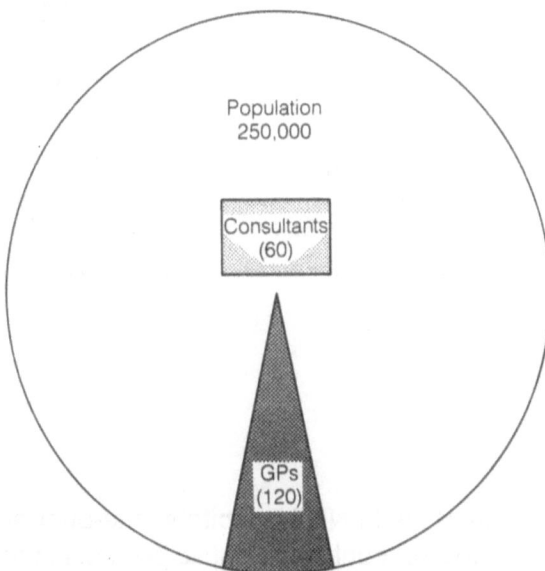

*Figure 1   NHS District of 250,000 with consultants and GPs
serving it*

Distributions of GPs and consultants

Since GPs now function as groups, of average four GPs per group,
there will be 25 GP units in the district. In the NHS there is one GP
to 2100 of the population and one consultant to 4200 of the population. The numbers of *consultants*, and their specialties in a district, are shown in Table 1.

Table 1   District: numbers of consultants and rate per population

Speciality	Consultants in a district	Consultants per population
General medicine	5	1:50,000
General surgery	5	1:50,000
OBG	3	1:80,000
Orthopaedics and trauma	4	1:62,500
Psychiatry	6	1:40,000
Paediatrics	3	1:80,000
Ophthalmology	2	1:125,000
Ear, nose and throat surgery	2	1:125,000
Geriatrics	2	1:125,000
Anaesthesia	8	1:30,000
Pathology	7	1:35,000
Radiology	5	1:50,000
Dermatology	1	1:250,000
Chest diseases	1	1:250,000
Others	6	1:40,000
Total	60	1:4200

Source: *Health and Personal Social Services Statistics, for England*, 1982

MORTALITY

Where?

Two thirds of death now take place in NHS hospitals, one-quarter at home and one in ten 'elsewhere' such as in public places, in the street, in a nursing home or hospice (Figure 2). In the 1950s more than one-half of all deaths were at home.

Table 2   Place of death

Place of death	Percentage
Hospital	65
Home	25
Elsewhere (hospice, public places, streets, etc.)	10

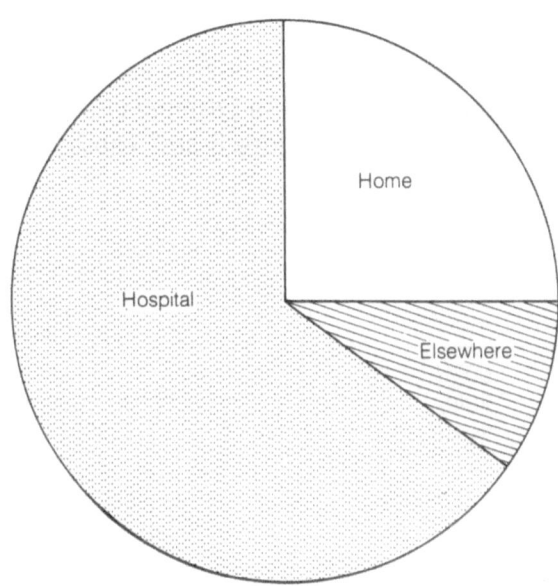

Figure 2 Place of death

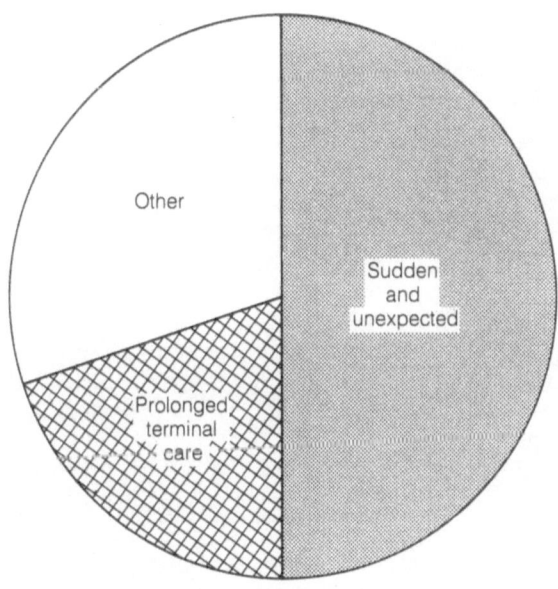

Figure 3 Type of death

How?

It is estimated that approximately one-half of deaths are sudden and unexpected, 20 per cent require long-term terminal care, and 30 per cent are somewhere in between (Figure 3 and Table 3).

Table 3   Type of death

Sudden and unexpected	50%
Prolonged terminal care	20%
Other	30%

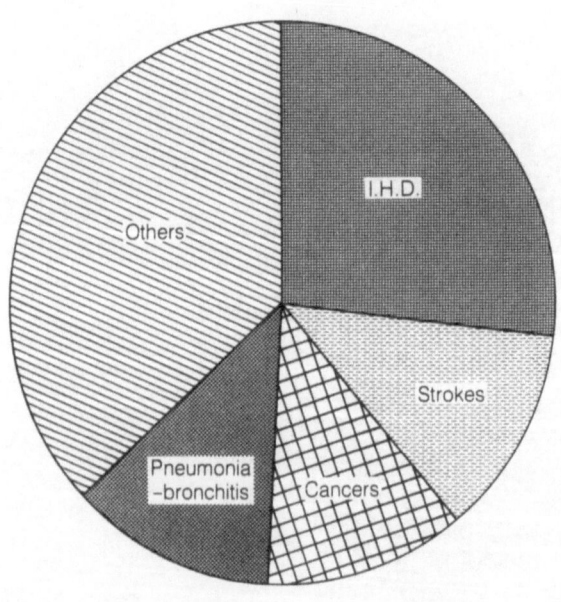

Figure 4   Causes of deaths in England (Health and Personal Social Services Statistics for England, *1982*)

What?

The causes of death (Figure 4 and Table 4) show the 'big 4' as ischaemic heart disease, strokes, cancers and pneumonia-bronchitis.

Table 4   Causes of Death in England (1980)

Cause	Percentage
IHD	27
Strokes	12
Cancers	12
Pneumonia–bronchitis	12
Accidents	3
High blood pressure	2
Suicide	<1 (0.9)
Chronic renal failure	<1 (0.9)
Diabetes	<1 (0.9)
Peptic ulcers	<1 (0.8)
Chronic rheumatic heart disease	<1 (0.6)
Congenital abnormalities	<1 (0.7)
Others	26
Numbers	544,000 deaths in England in 1980

Source: *Health and Personal Social Services Statistics for England*, 1982

Trends

Over the period 1968–1980 there were trends in standardized mortality ratios (SMRs) (Figure 5a–c).

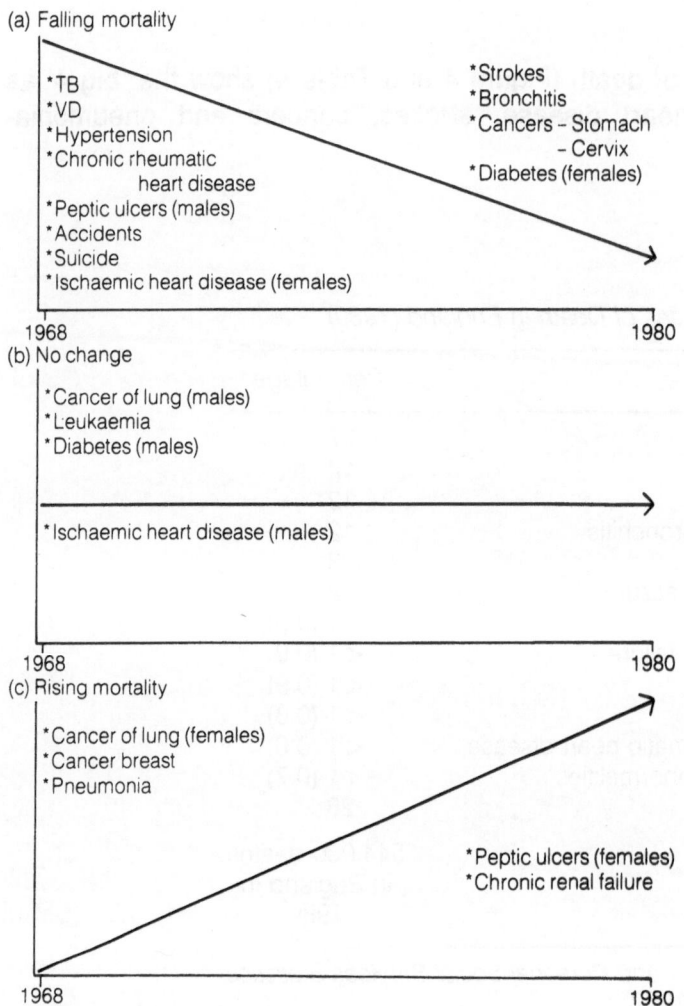

(a) Falling mortality

*TB
*VD
*Hypertension
*Chronic rheumatic
        heart disease
*Peptic ulcers (males)
*Accidents
*Suicide
*Ischaemic heart disease (females)

*Strokes
*Bronchitis
*Cancers – Stomach
        – Cervix
*Diabetes (females)

1968   1980

(b) No change

*Cancer of lung (males)
*Leukaemia
*Diabetes (males)

*Ischaemic heart disease (males)

1968   1980

(c) Rising mortality

*Cancer of lung (females)
*Cancer breast
*Pneumonia

*Peptic ulcers (females)
*Chronic renal failure

1968   1980

Figure 5   SMRs 1968–1980, England

Age

Figure 6 shows the age–sex proportions of selected causes of death in 1980.

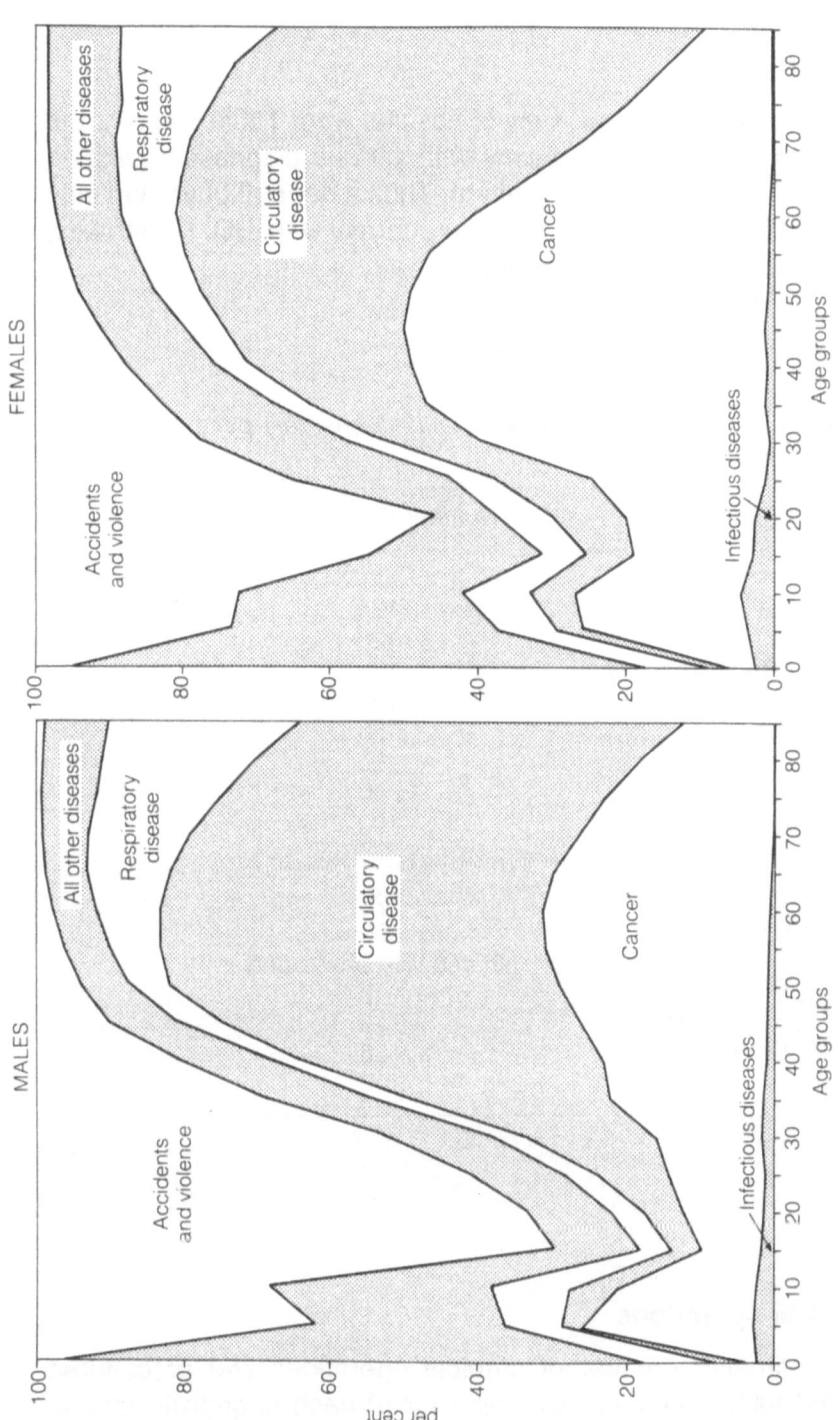

Figure 6   Selected causes of death, by sex and age, 1980 (Social Trends, *1982, Chart 7.4*)

MORBIDITY

To give a 'personalized' view of hospital work Table 5 shows the estimated numbers of persons with various diagnoses admitted under the care of each consultant. Thus a general physician may expect 125 persons under his care each year with IHD, 120 strokes, 100 cases of pneumonia–bronchitis, etc.

Table 5   Annual inpatients (deaths and discharges) per consultant, in various specialties

Specialty	Number IPs per year
Medical	
IHD	125
Strokes	120
Pneumonia–bronchitis	100
Depression	100
Asthma	50
Cancer of lung	50
Diabetes (new)	40
Parasuicide	100
Surgical	
'Acute abdomen'	125
Peptic ulcers	60
	(shared with physicians)
Cancer of breast	40
Cancer of bowel	15
Gall bladder	35
Fibroids	100

Surgical operations

The estimated number of surgical operations and procedures carried out by, or under the supervision of, each surgeon (in various specialties) are shown in Table 6.

Table 6   Estimated annual numbers of surgical operations per consultant surgeon at a district general hospital

Surgical operation/procedure	Numbers per consultant per year
'D and C'	200
'Ts and As'	200
Cataract	100
Fractures	100
Hysterectomy	100
Termination of pregnancy	100
Cystoscopy	80
Appendicectomy	70
Inguinal hernia	60
Breast	50
Squint	50
Laparascopic sterilization	50
Arthroplasty	45
Gall bladder	40
Prostatectomy	30
Circumcision	25
Perineal repair	20
Colectomy	15
Thyroid	10

Hospital outpatients

The likely diagnostic composition of outpatients in selected specialties is shown in Table 7. Note the high proportions of 'NAD' (nothing abnormal detected).

General practice

Morbidity in general practice is different in degree and content from that in hospitals. The emphasis is on minor and chronic conditions (Figure 7 and Table 8).

Table 7   Outpatients: composition of selected special-ties

Specialty and main diagnoses	Percentage of total for each specialty
General medical	
Cardiovascular	17
Endocrine	12
Rheumatic	13
Gastro-intestinal	10
CNS	7
'NAD'	26
Other	15
General surgical	
New growths	14
Herniae	13
Genito-urinary	13
Gastro-intestinal	13
Varicose veins	7
Piles	4
'NAD'	16
Other	20
Gynaecological	
Infections	15
Prolapse	14
Fibroids and new growths	13
'NAD'	18
Other	40

Table 8   General practice morbidity – severity of disease

Severity	Percentage
Minor – brief self-limiting	65
Chronic – long-lasting and non-curable	20
Major – acute and life-threatening	15

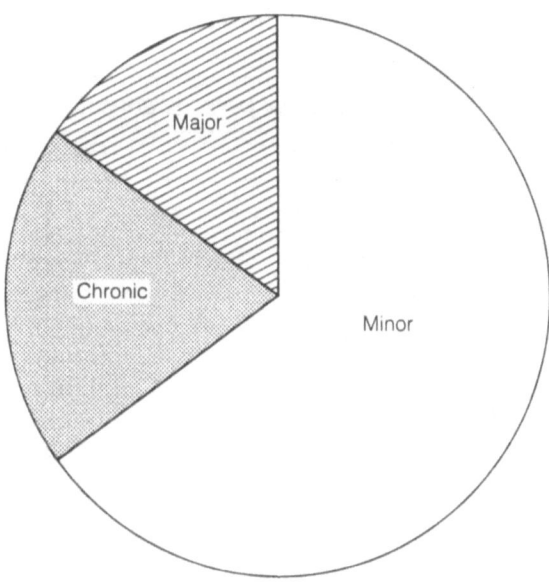

Figure 7   General practice morbidity – severity of disease

Minor, chronic and major disease

Tables 9–12 demonstrate the annual numbers of persons consulting in general practice. The numbers are for a GP with 2500 patients and for a group of 10,000 patients.

Table 9   Minor conditions in general practice: annual person consulting rates

	Annual persons consulting	
Condition-group	Per 10,000	Per 2500
Upper respiratory infections	2400	600
Skin disorders	1400	350
Psycho-emotional problems	1000	250
Minor accidents	1000	250
Gastro-intestinal conditions	800	200
Rheumatics	600	150
'Symptoms'	1500	375

Table 10   Specific minor conditions in general practice: annual person consulting rates

Condition	Annual persons consulting	
	Per 10,000	Per 2500
Acute throat infections	400	100
Lacerations	400	100
Eczema–dermatitis	400	100
Acute otitis media	300	75
Ear wax	200	50
Urinary tract infections	200	50
Acute backache	200	50
Vaginal discharge	120	30
Migraine	100	25
Hay fever	100	25
Vertigo–dizziness	80	20
Hernia	60	15
Piles	60	15

Table 11   Chronic disease in general practice: annual person consulting rates

Condition	Annual persons consulting	
	Per 10,000	Per 2500
High blood pressure	1000	250
Chronic rheumatism (arthritis)	400	100
Chronic psychiatric	400	100
IHD	200	50
Obesity	200	50
Congestive cardiac failure	160	40
Anaemia	120	30
Cancers (under care)	120	30
Asthma	120	30
Diabetes	120	30
Varicose veins	120	30
Peptic ulcers	100	25
Strokes	80	20
Thyroid disorders	40	10
Epilepsy	40	10
Multiple sclerosis	12	3
Parkinsonism	12	3
Chronic renal failure	2	less than 1

Table 12 Major disease in general practice: annual person consulting rate

Condition	Annual persons consulting	
	Per 10,000	Per 2500
Acute bronchitis	400	100
Pneumonia	80	20
Severe depression	40	10
(Parasuicide)	(16)	(4)
(Suicide)	(1)	(1 every 4 years)
Acute myocardial infarction	40	10
(Sudden death)	(20)	(5)
Acute strokes	20	5
All new cancers	20	5
Acute appendicitis	15	5

COMMENT

- In a *district* of 250,000 persons there are 120 general practitioners and 60 consultants.
- There is approximately 1 *GP* to 2100 persons and 1 *consultant* to 4200 persons.
- Of the ½ million *deaths* annually, 27 per cent are caused by ischaemic heart disease, 12 per cent by strokes, 11 per cent by cancers and 12 per cent by bronchitis–pneumonia.
- Sixty-five per cent of *deaths* take place in hospital, 25 per cent at home and 10 per cent elsewhere.
- Fifty per cent of *deaths* are sudden and unexpected and 20 per cent terminal and prolonged.
- The most frequent conditions in *hospital wards* are ischaemic heart disease, strokes, pneumonia–bronchitis and depression; 'acute abdomens', fibroids and peptic ulcers.
- The most frequent *surgical operations* are 'D & C' and 'Ts and As', followed by cataract removal, fractures, hysterectomy and termination of pregnancy.

- In over 20 per cent of *new outpatient consultations* no organic disease is detected.
- In *general practice* 65 per cent of work is with minor conditions, 20 per cent with chronic disorders and 15 per cent with major life-threatening situations.
- The bulk of *medical work* in hospitals and general practice is with 'common diseases that commonly occur'. These tend to be medically mundane (to the doctor).
- The *medical services* must be geared to provide most resources to care for common conditions.

CHAPTER 4

SOCIAL PATHOLOGIES

CIGARETTE SMOKING

Between 1972 and 1980 the proportion of smokers in all groups fell, but especially among professionals. Average weekly cigarette consumption in smokers in 1980 was 124 (18 per day) for men and 102 (15 per day) for women (Figures 1 and 2).

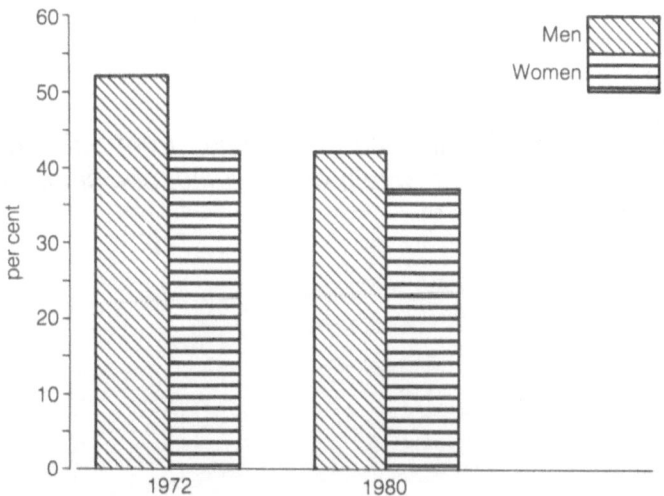

Figure 1   Cigarette smoking: percentages of all persons smoking (Social Trends, *1983, Table 7.12)*

Drugs

Notified addicts have increased steadily since 1971 (Figure 3). Most are men. There are many other addicts who have not been notified.

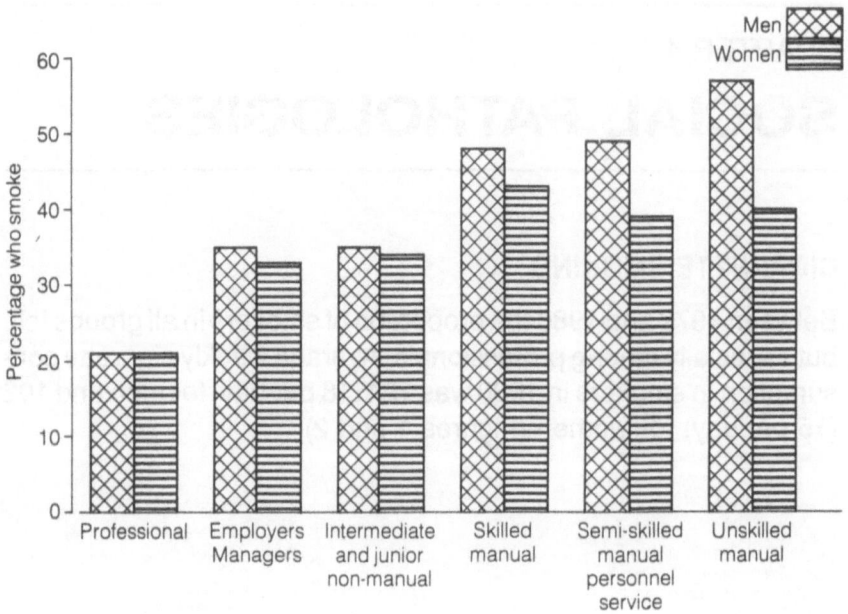

Figure 2   Cigarette smoking in men and women from different socioeconomic groups in Great Britain during 1980: percentages (Social Trends, *1983, Table 7.12*)

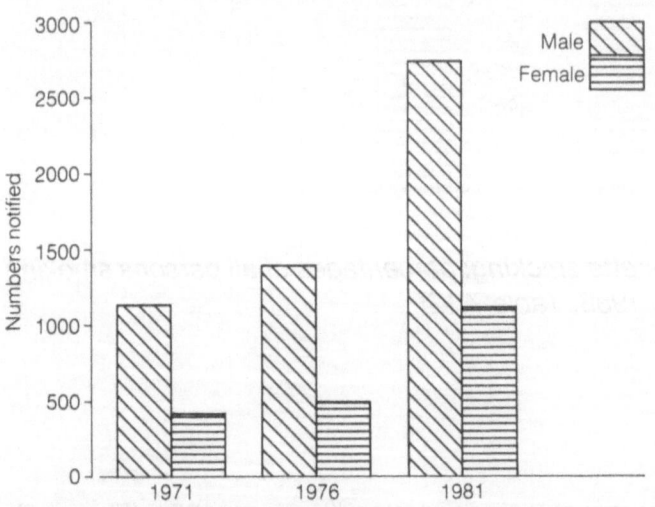

Figure 3   Notified drug addicts among men and women, United Kingdom (Social Trends, *1983, Table 7.11*)

Alcohol

Heavy drinkers are twice as prevalent in men under the age of 44 than in older men, and about one-third of men describe themselves as frequent light drinkers (Figure 4).

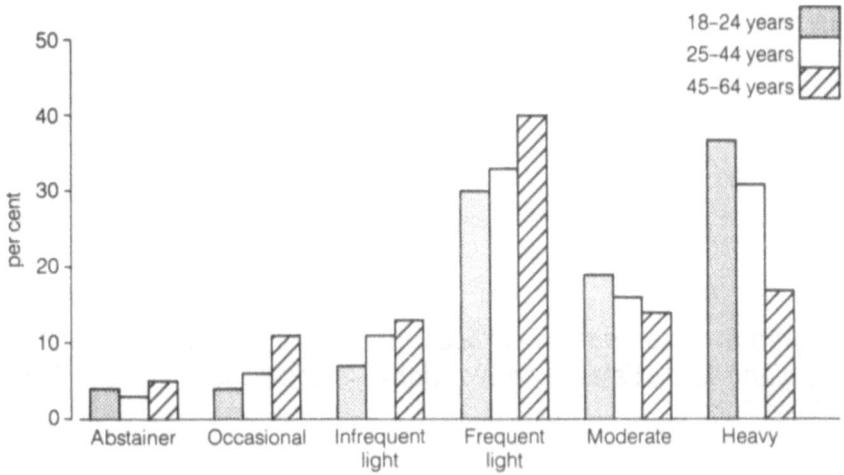

*Figure 4   Drinking habits in men in different age groups, 1980, Great Britain (*Social Trends, *1983, Table 7.8)*

Deaths from cirrhosis of the liver

Deaths from cirrhosis of the liver have increased since 1961, especially in Scotland (Figure 5).

Accidents and alcohol consumption

Alcohol is a significant contributory factor in road traffic accidents. Figure 6 shows that 30 per cent of drivers and pedestrians killed had blood alcohol levels above 80 mg/100 ml. Figure 7 shows that in 10 per cent of all road traffic accidents alcohol was a contributory factor.

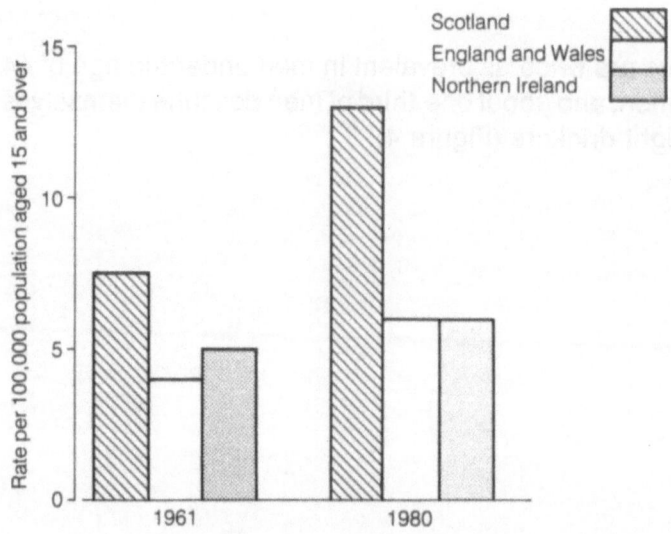

Figure 5   Deaths from cirrhosis of the liver in men in Scotland, England and Wales, and Northern Ireland (Social Trends, *1983,* Chart 7.9)

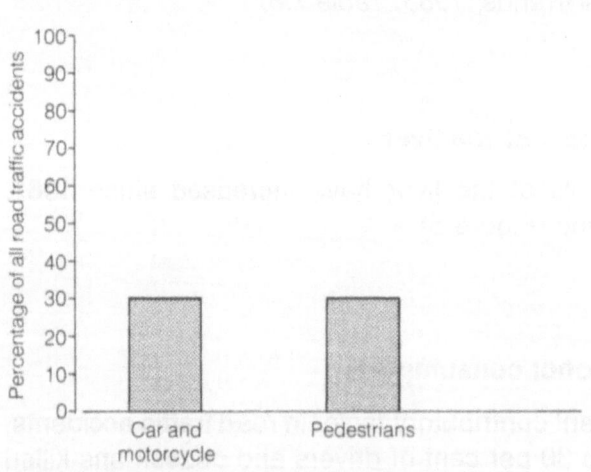

Figure 6   Blood alcohol levels above 80 mg/100 ml, Great Britain, 1979–1980 (Br. Med. J. *(1982), 284, 520)*

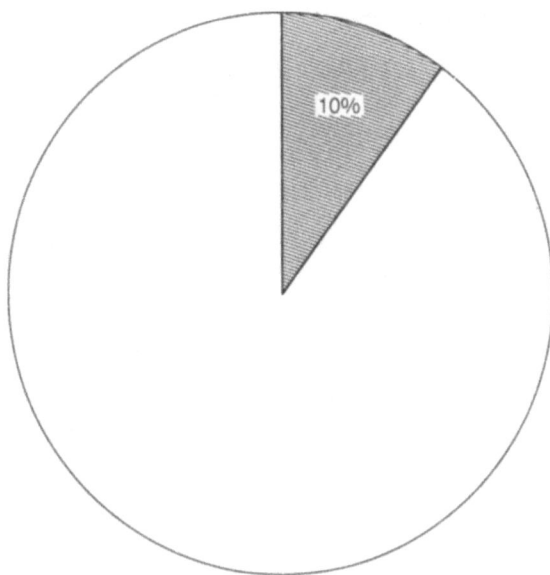

*Figure 7   Alcohol as a contributory factor in all road traffic acci-
dents in Great Britain, including damage-only accidents, 1979–
1980 (Br. Med. J. (1982), 284, 520)*

Road traffic accidents

Total road casualties have been falling slightly since 1966 despite
a 50 per cent increase of road motor vehicles with licences
(Figure 8).

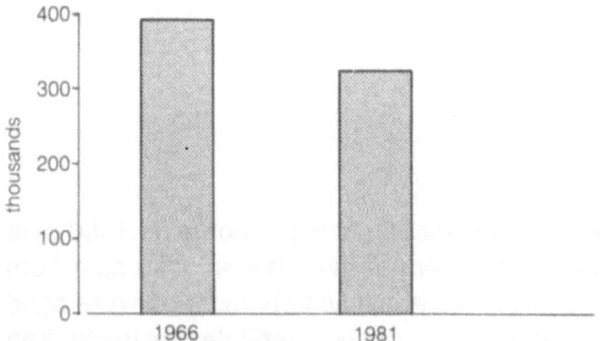

*Figure 8   Total road casualties in thousands, Great Britain (Social
Trends, 1983, Table 7.15)*

Casualty rates for different road users

Cars are safer than cycles or motor bikes (Figure 9).

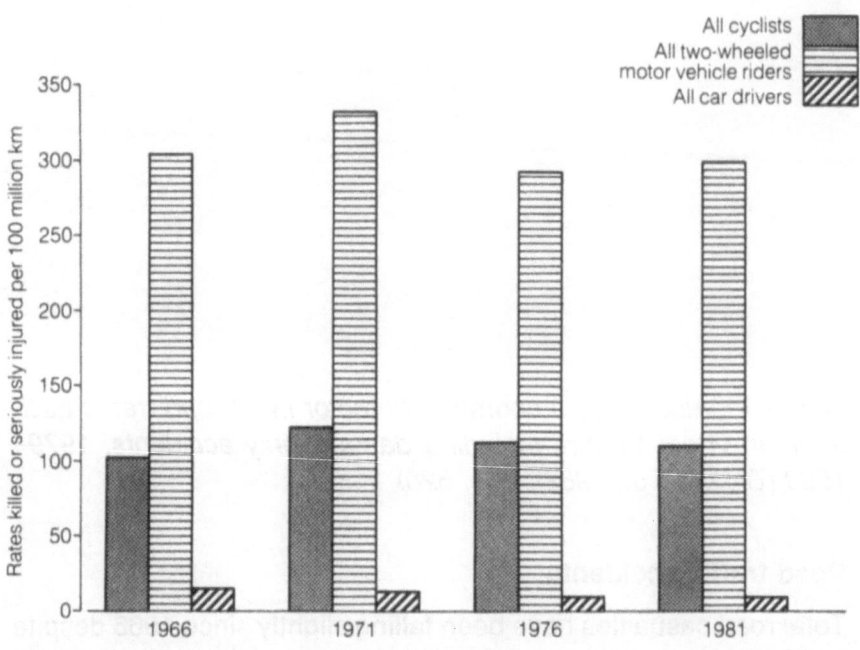

*Figure 9   Casualty rates for different road users, **Great Britain,
1966–1981** (Social Trends, 1983, Table 7.15)*

Accidents in the home

Old persons have most of the accidents in the home. In 1980 over
half the males, and three-quarters of the females, who died from
accidents in the home or in residential accommodation were aged
65 or over. The commonest cause of accidental deaths in children
was suffocating, in the 15–44 age group poisoning, and in the
over-45s falls (Figure 10).

54   SOCIAL PATHOLOGIES

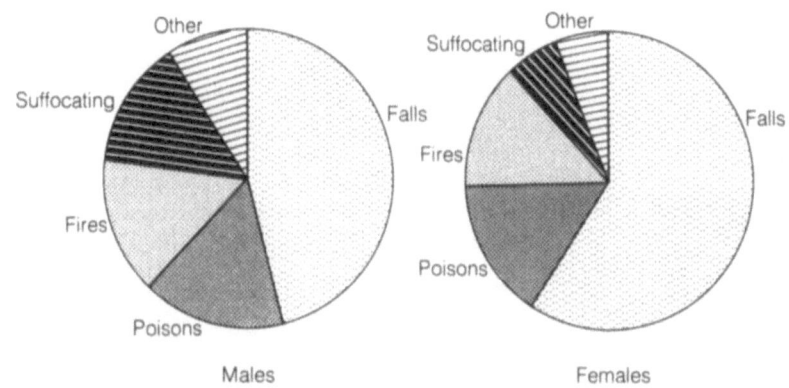

Figure 10   Deaths from accidents in the home, Great Britain, 1980
(Social Trends, *1983, Table 7.16)*

DISABLED AND HANDICAPPED

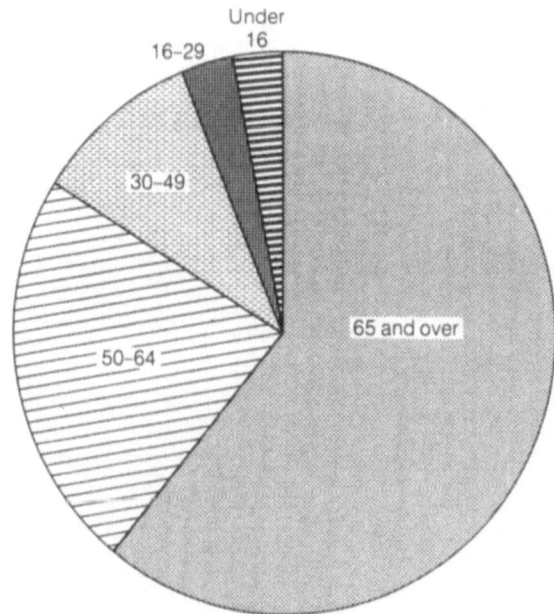

*Figure 11   Handicap by age, England, 1981 (*Health and Personal
Social Statistics, *1982, Table 7.12)*

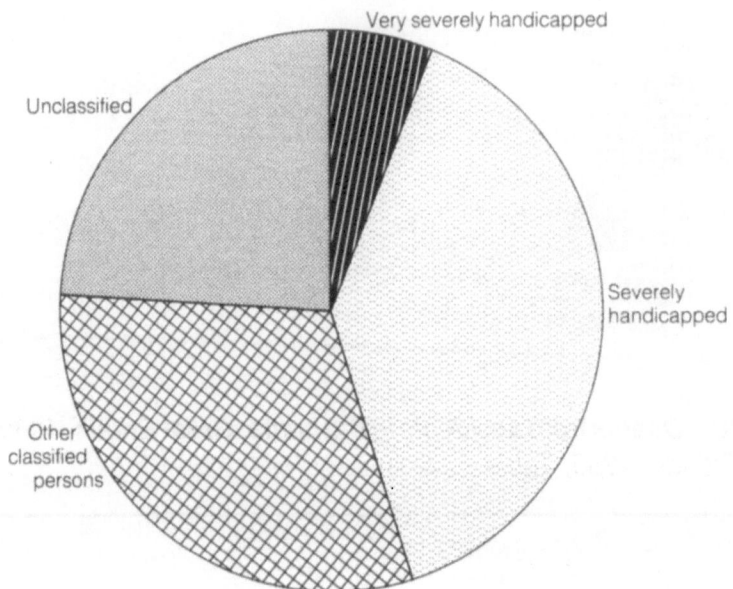

Figure 12   Handicap by severity, England, 1981 (Health and Personal Social Services Statistics, *1982, Table 7.12)*

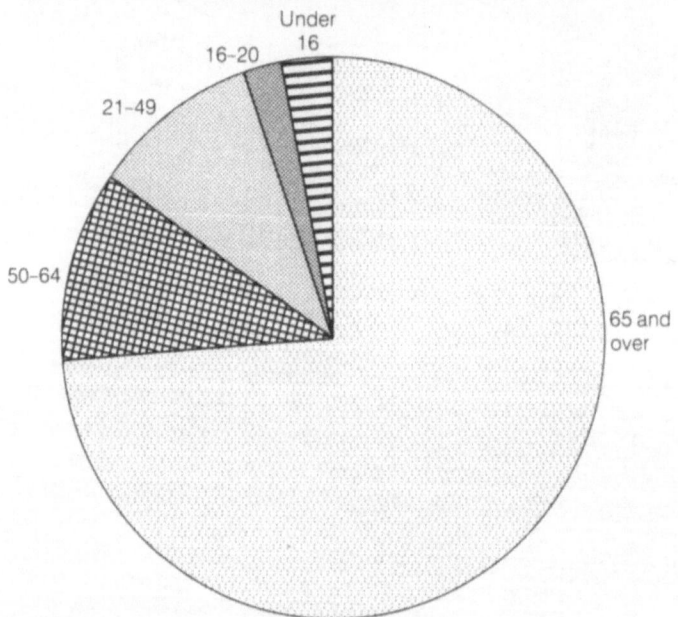

Figure 13   Blindness by age, England, 1980 (Health and Personal Social Statistics, *1982, Table 7.12)*

56   SOCIAL PATHOLOGIES

An estimated 500,000 people have been issued with an orange badge for parking concessions in the United Kingdom. In 1980 more than 1 million were registered substantially and permanently handicapped. Figure 11 shows the age distributions and Figure 12 the severity.

There were 107,800 registered blind in England in 1980. An additional 51,400 were registered partially sighted (Figure 13).

Deafness

A total of 29,700 people were registered deaf in 1980 and 35,100 people were registered hard-of-hearing in 1980. Most were over 65.

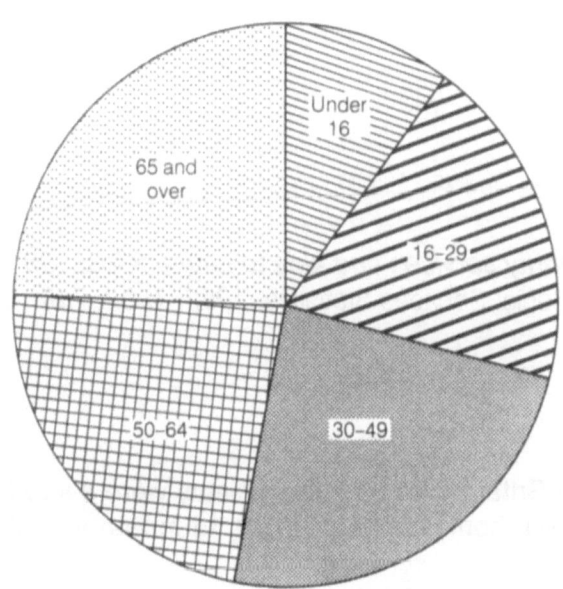

Figure 14   Deafness by age, England, 1980 (Health and Personal Social Statistics, *1982, Table 7.12*)

LOCAL AUTHORITY SERVICES

Aids and holidays

Local authorities provided aids and benefits to half a million persons in 1981 (Figure 15).

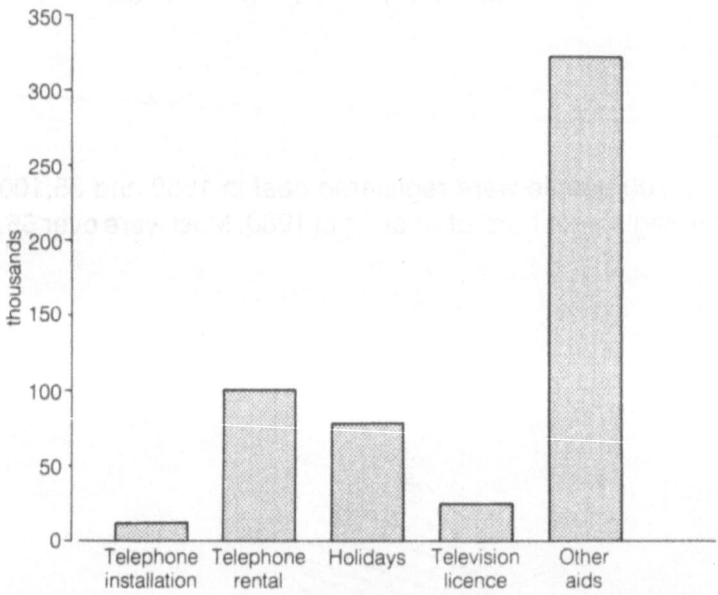

Figure 15   Local authority services and aids to households, 1981
(Health and Personal Social Services Statistics, *1982, Table 7.8*)

Meals services

In 1980–1981 in Great Britain over 30 million meals were served to the elderly in their own homes, and a further 18 million at day centres.

Home help services

Staff and services almost doubled between 1971 and 1981 (Figure 16).

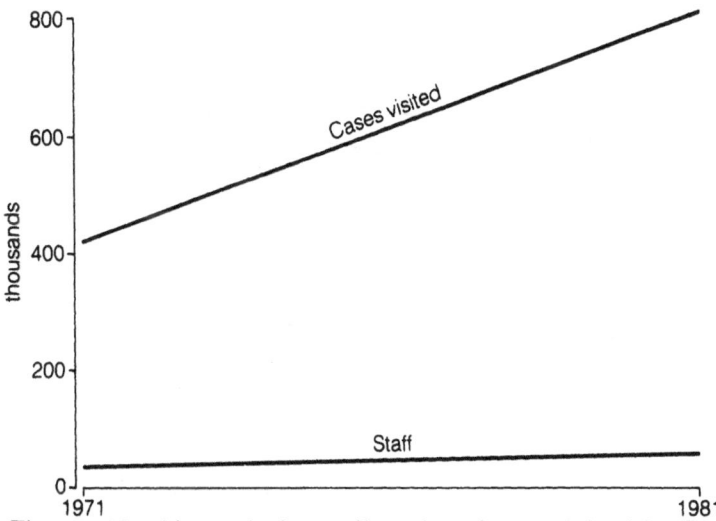

Figure 16 Home help staff and patients visited in England and Wales between 1971 and 1980 (Social Trends, *1982, Table 13.20)*

Local authority accommodation

In 1981, 170,300 people over 65 were in residential accommodation for the elderly (Figure 17). The numbers of local authority homes, private and voluntary (nursing) homes for the elderly have also increased (Figure 18).

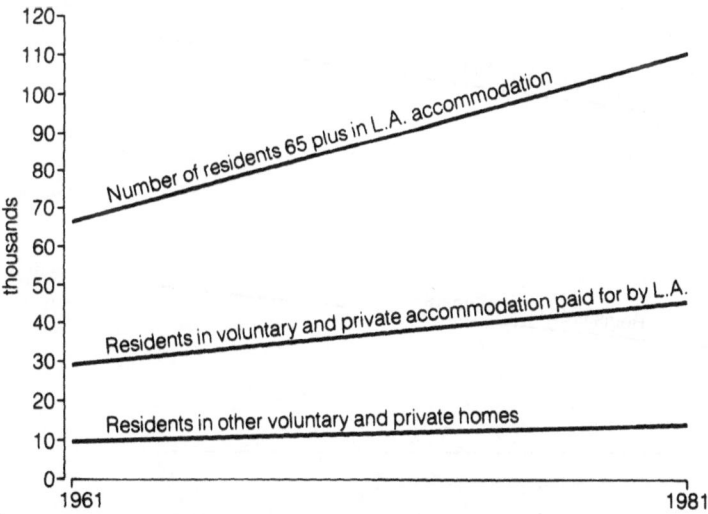

Figure 17 Residential accommodation for the elderly in England and Wales (Social Trends, *1983, Table 7.29)*

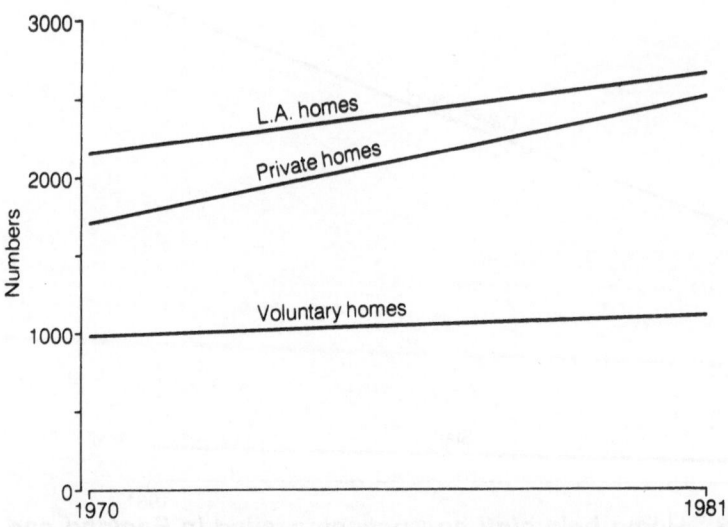

Figure 18   Numbers of local authority and private homes for the elderly and physically handicapped in England (Health and Personal Social Services Statistics, *1982, Tables 7.1 and 7.2*)

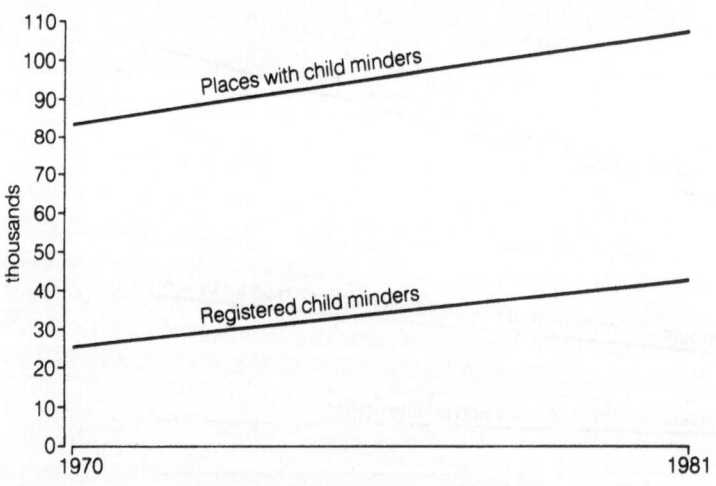

Figure 19   Registered child minders in England (Health and Personal Social Services Statistics, *1982, Table 7.6*)

Child minders and nurseries

More preschool children are receiving day care outside the home (Figures 19 and 20).

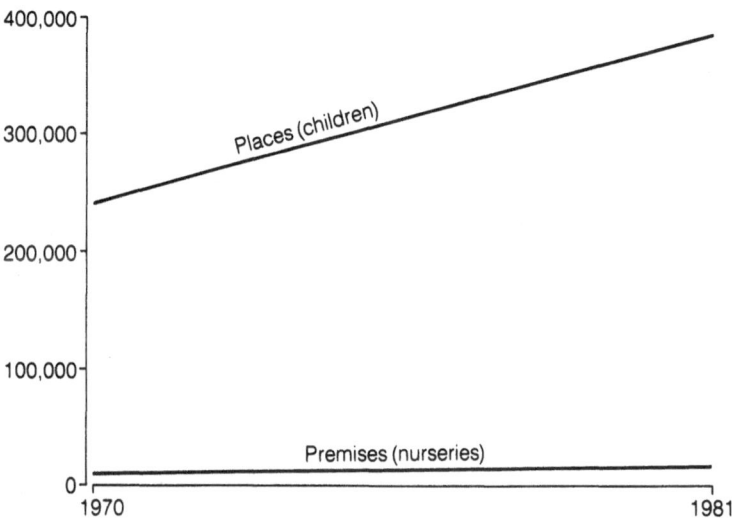

Figure 20 **Registered nurseries in England** (Health and Personal Social Services Statistics, *1982, Table 7.6)*

Children in care

A total of 100,200 children were in care in England and Wales in 1980 (Figure 21). The reasons for the children being taken into care are shown in Figure 22.

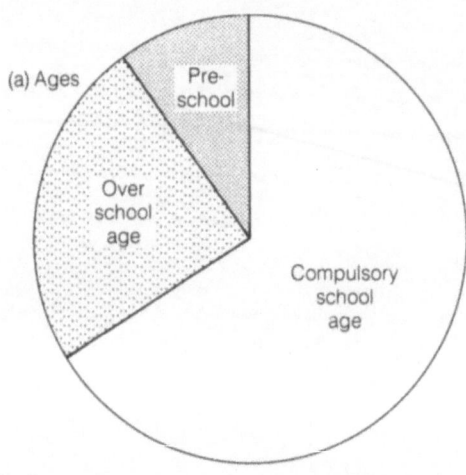

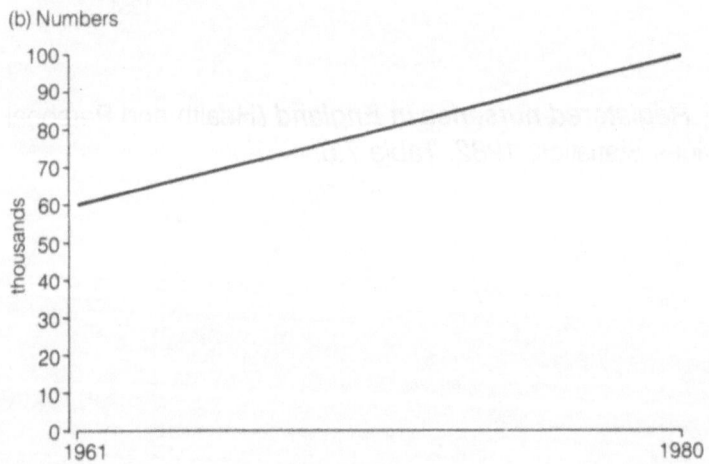

Figure 21   Children in care, England (Health and Personal Social Services Statistics, *1982, Table 7.9*)

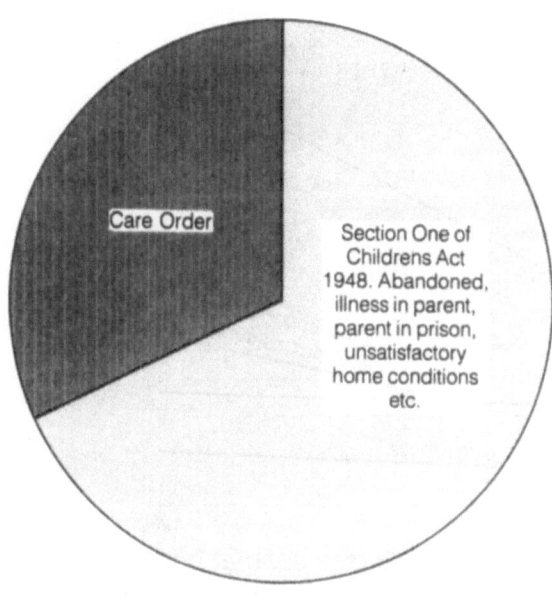

Within the pie chart:
Care Order

Section One of
Childrens Act
1948. Abandoned,
illness in parent,
parent in prison,
unsatisfactory
home conditions
etc.

Figure 22   The circumstances in which children came into care in England in 1980 (Health and Personal Social Services Statistics, *1982, Table 7.9)*

SEXUALLY TRANSMITTED DISEASES

Sexually transmitted diseases have been increasing sharply, apart from syphilis which decreased from 12,931 cases in 1949 to 4059 in 1980 (Figure 23).

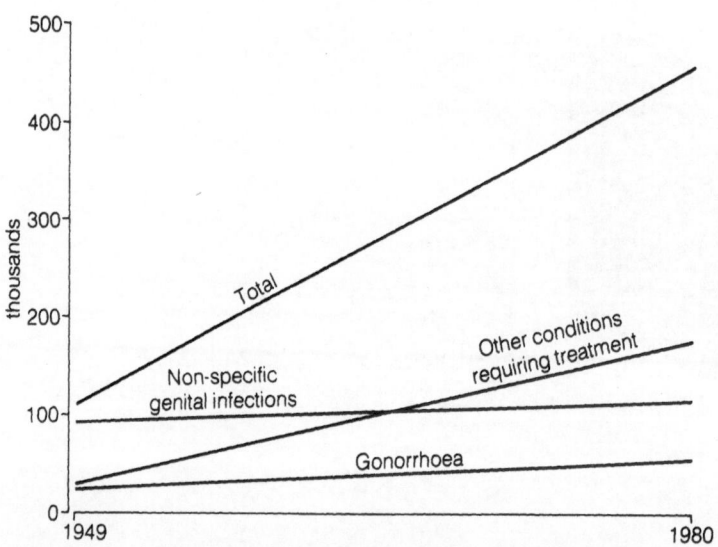

Figure 23   Sexually transmitted diseases seen at hospital clinics between 1949 and 1980, England (Health and Personal Social Services Statistics, *1982, Table 11.5)*

Legal abortions

Between 1971 and 1981 the total number of abortions in England and Wales increased by 36 per cent (Figure 24).

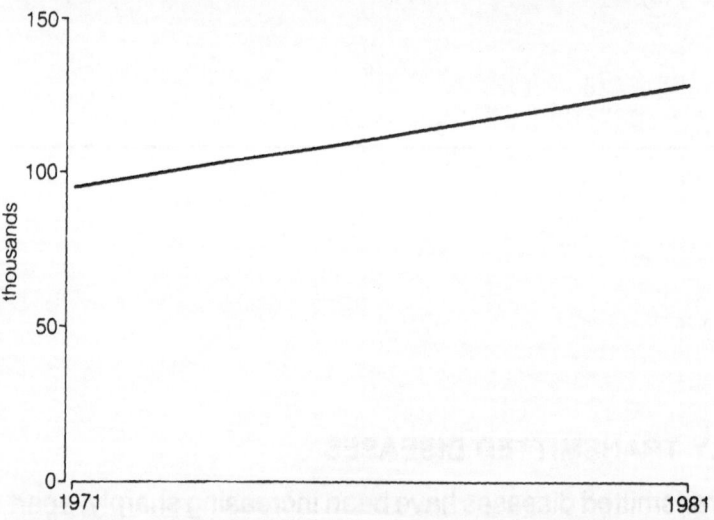

*Figure 24   Total number of abortions to residents, England and Wales (*Social Trends, *1983, Table 2.22)*

64   SOCIAL PATHOLOGIES

Place of abortion

Private hospitals and clinics increased their contribution to the total number of abortions notified (Figure 25). The proportion of abortions carried out on single women has been increasing (Figure 26). Ninety-eight per cent of abortions are carried out under two of the four legal grounds for abortion (Figure 27).

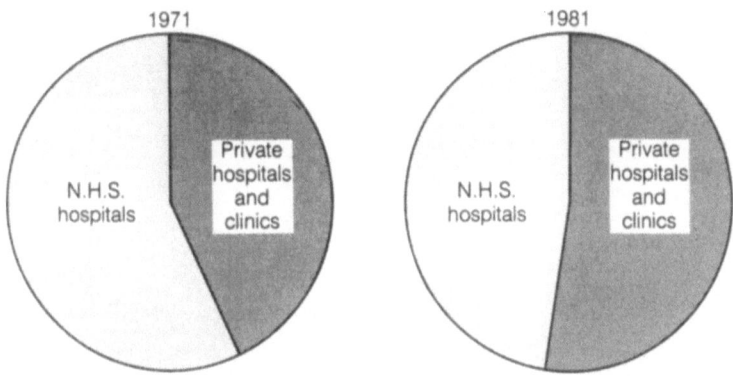

Figure 25   Place of abortion (Social Trends, *1983, Table 2.22*)

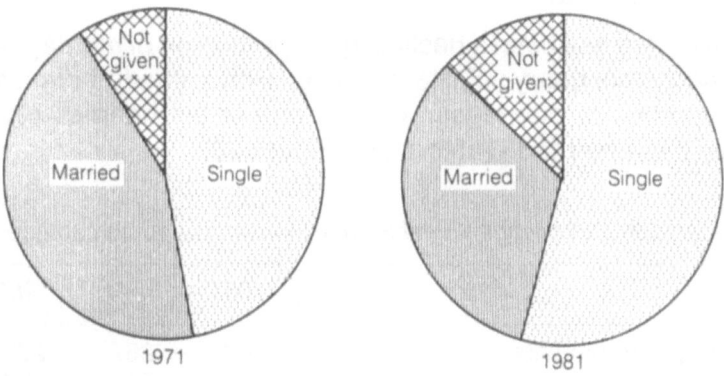

Figure 26   Abortions: single and married women (Social Trends, *1983, Table 2.22*)

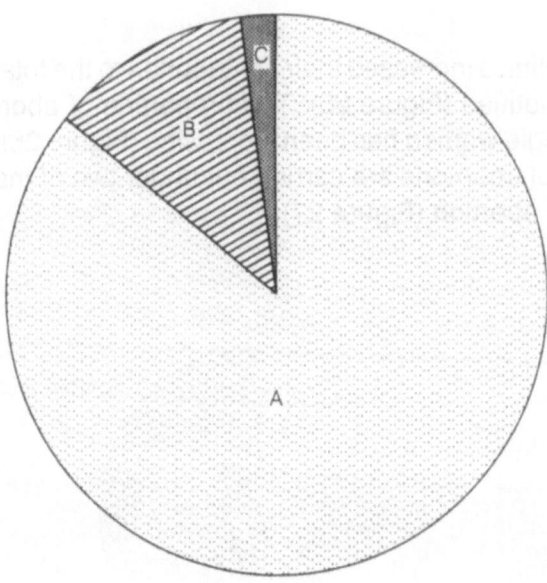

A. Risk of injury to mental/physical health of woman
B. Risk of injury to mental/physical health of existing children
C. Others

*Figure 27 Grounds for abortion, 1981 (*Social Trends, *1983, Table 2.22)*

Marriage and divorce

Since 1961 there has been a decline in the proportion of marriages in which bachelors marry spinsters coupled with a steady increase in the proportion of marriages in which one or both parties had previously been married (Table 1 and Figure 28).

Table 1   Marriage and divorce, Great Britain: thousands and percentages

	1961	1971	1980
First marriage both partners	331	357	270
Total marriages	387	447	409
Remarriage as a percentage of all marriages	15%	20%	34%

Source: *Social Trends*, 1983, Table 2.12

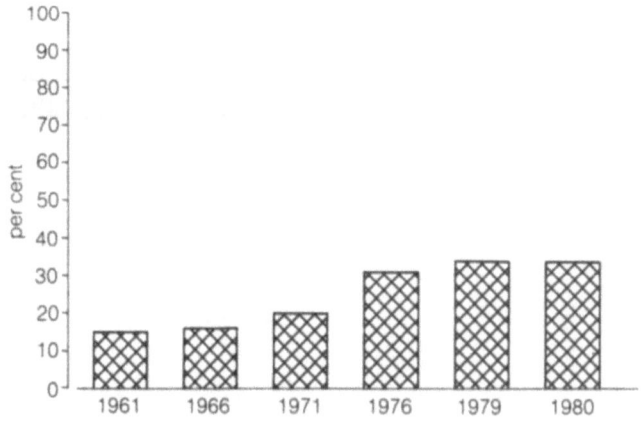

Figure 28 *Remarriage as percentage of all marriages, United Kingdom, 1961–1980* (Social Trends, *1983, Table 2.12*)

Divorce

In 1981 a total of 157,000 decrees were made absolute in the United Kingdom, which is almost double the number in 1971 when the Divorce Reform Act came into force (Figure 29).

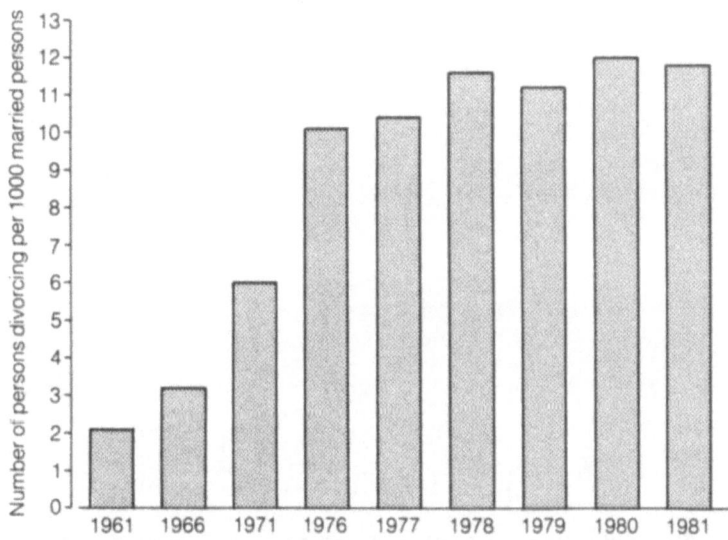

Figure 29 *The number of persons divorcing per 1000 married people, United Kingdom (*Social Trends, *1983, Table 2.15)*

Divorce by duration of marriages

The proportion of divorces in Great Britain occurring within 4 years of marriage has increased between 1961 and 1981 (Figure 30).

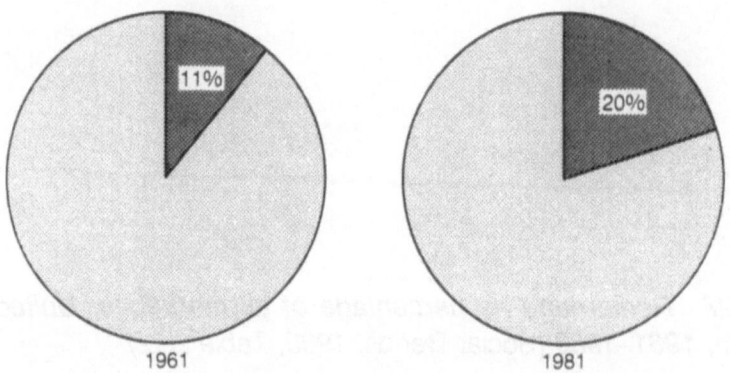

Figure 30   Divorce within 4 years of marriage (Social Trends, *1983,* Table 2.16)

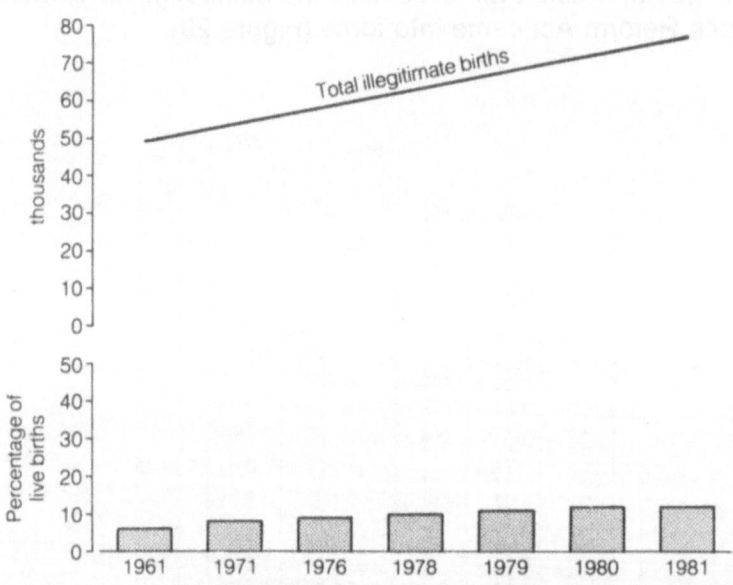

Figure 31   Total illegitimate births absolute and as a percentage of total live births, England and Wales (Social Trends, *1983, Table 2.19)*

Illegitimate births

About 90 per cent of couples in their first marriages have children, but the number and proportion of illegitimate births continues to rise despite easier contraception (Figure 31).

Suicides

Total suicides represent less than 1 per cent of total deaths each year in the United Kingdom, but this proportion is 12 per cent in those aged 25–29 (Figure 32). Suicide is commoner in men in all age groups, and rates increase with age. Suicide is commonest in the 65–74 age group in women (Figure 33).

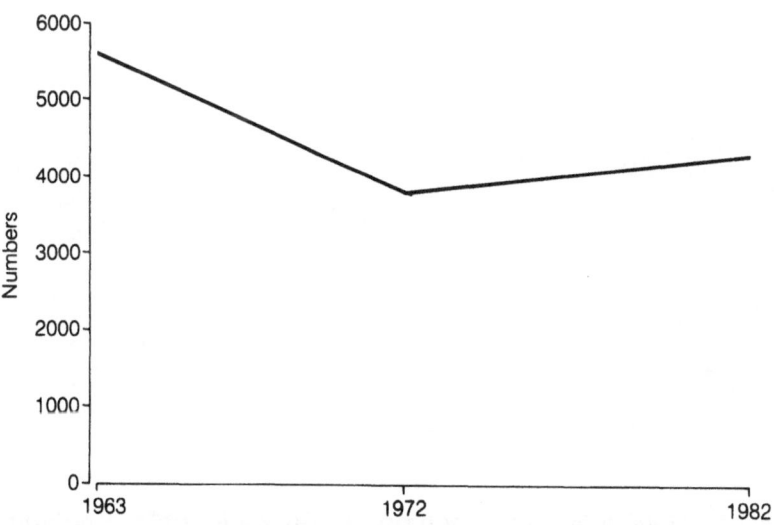

Figure 32   Suicides 1963–1980, England and Wales

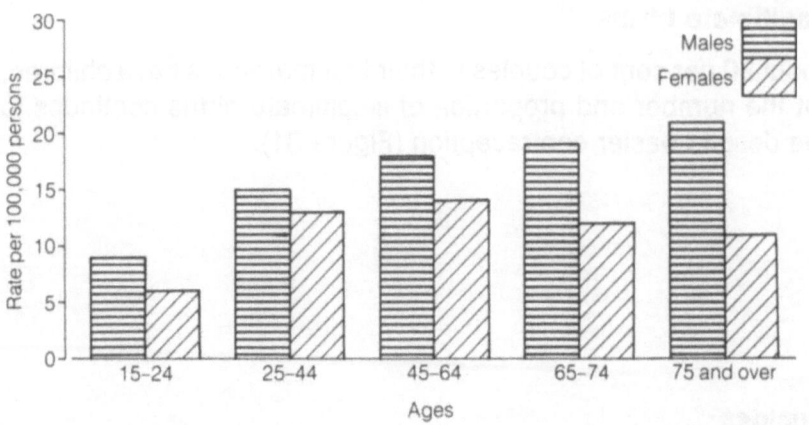

Figure 33   Suicides by sex and age, United Kingdom, 1980 (Social Trends, 1983, Chart 7.3)

Crime

Almost 3 million notifiable offences were recorded by the police in England and Wales in 1981, an increase of 10 per cent over 1980. Theft, and the handling of stolen goods, accounted for just over half of all offences recorded, and burglary for a further quarter (Figure 34).

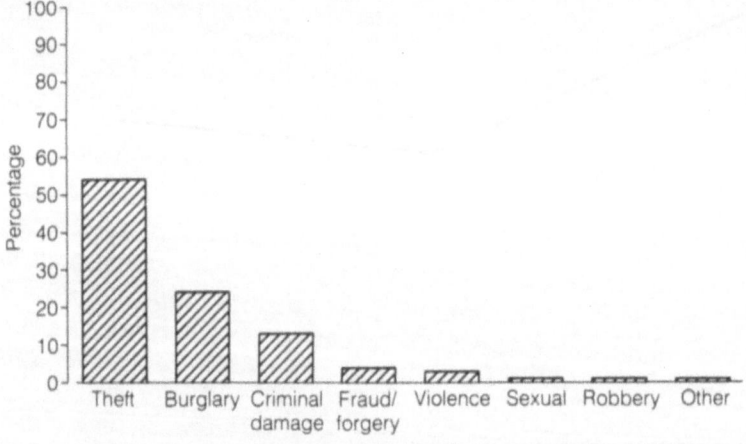

Figure 34   Notifiable crime by type of offence in 1981, England and Wales (total 2,963,800) (Social Trends, 1983, Table 12.1)

COMMENT

- Cigarette smoking is falling and particularly in professional classes.
- Smokers' daily consumption is 18 cigarettes for men and 15 for women.
- Drug addiction has increased; most addicts have never been notified.
- Alcohol – heaviest drinkers are males under 45.
- Alcohol – in 30 per cent of road traffic accidents blood alcohol was above limit.
- Road traffic accidents have fallen in spite of more cars.
- Disabled – more than 1 million.
- Local authorities provide aids and services for more than ½ million.
- Sexually transmitted diseases are increasing.
- Abortions are increasing.
- First marriages decreasing.
- Divorces increasing.
- Illegitimate births increasing.
- Crime increasing.
- Suicides decreasing.

CHAPTER 5

INEQUALITIES IN HEALTH CORRELATES OF SOCIAL CLASS

Despite 30 years of the National Health Service, manual workers and their families still are prone to die younger and have more ill health than professional people. Indeed there is evidence that the gap between the two social groups is increasing.

THE SOCIAL CLASS STRUCTURE OF THE COMMUNITY

Since 1875 the Registrar General has divided the population into broad occupational groups or classes based on job income and status. Married women assume their husband's social class (Figure 1).

Table 1   The Registrar General's social class classification

Class	Occupation	Percentage
I	Professional – accountant, lawyer, doctor	5
II	Intermediate – manager, school teacher	18
III N	Skilled non-manual – clerical worker, secretary, shop assistant	12 ⎫
III M	Skilled manual – bus driver, butcher, coal miner, carpenter	38 ⎬ 50
IV	Partly skilled – agricultural worker, bus conductor, postman	18
V	Unskilled – labourer, cleaner	9

Source: *Inequalities in Health: the Black Report*. Edited by Townsend, P. and Davidson, N. (1982). London: Penguin, p. 48

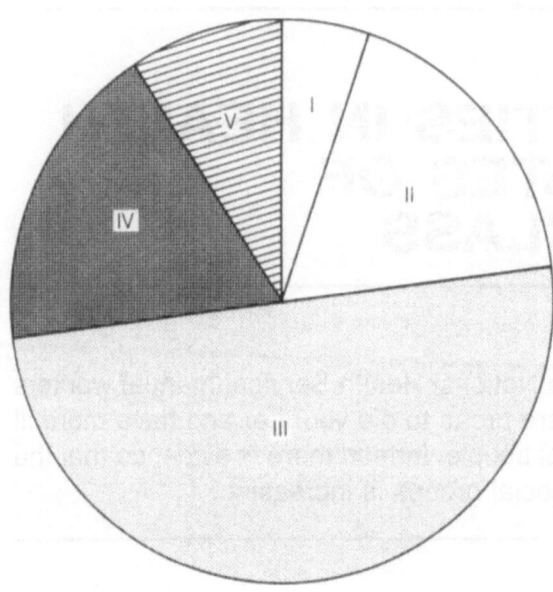

Figure 1   The Registrar General's social class classification

DEATH RATES AND SOCIAL CLASS

In all social classes males have higher mortality rates. A progressive rise in mortality rates occurs from class I to class V in both sexes (Figure 2). Health differences between classes can be traced through all stages of life. A child born into a family at the bottom of the social scale is twice as likely to die at birth or in the first few months of life. For every child from the professional class who dies before reaching his first birthday we can expect two deaths in the skilled manual class and four deaths in the lowest social class. Only at the age group 5–19 years is there no excess mortality in lower social classes.

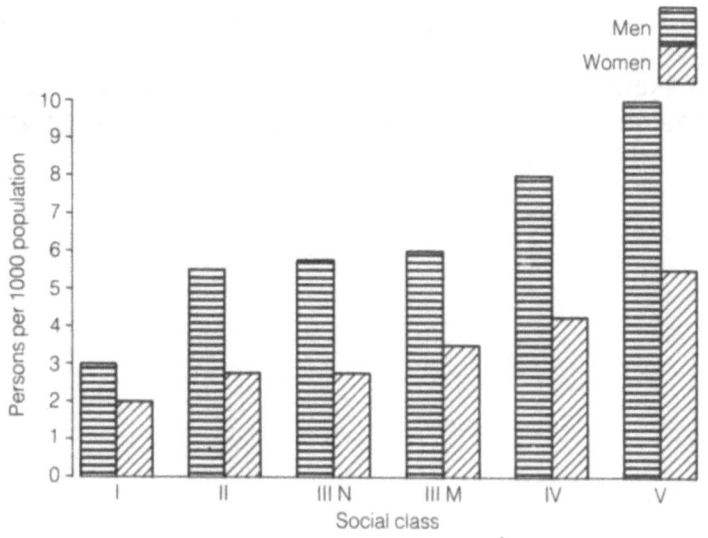

Figure 2 *Death rates by social class and sex (15–64) years, England and Wales, 1971 (Townsend and Davidson, 1982, p. 57)*

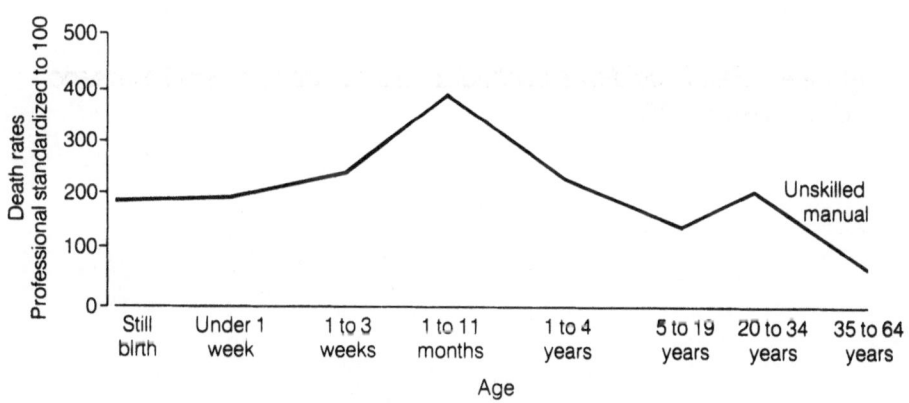

Figure 3 *Death rates of unskilled manual workers as a percentage of death rates among professional workers by age groups, 1971–1972 (Townsend and Davidson, 1982)*

Accidents account for nearly one-third of all deaths under 14 years. However, a boy from the family of an unskilled worker is ten times more likely to die by fire, fall or drowning than a boy from a professional family and seven times more likely to be knocked down and killed by a car.

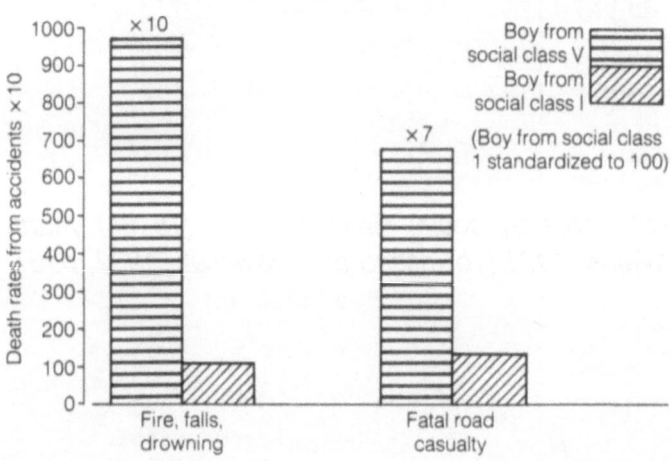

Figure 4 *Fatal accidents in childhood and social class (Townsend and Davidson, 1982)*

Table 2 illustrates a marked gradient from sedentary non-manual to heavy unskilled manual and is accompanied by wide variations between mortality rates for specific occupations within each occupational class.

Table 2 Mortality by occupation unit – men, 15–64

Occupation unit	Direct age-standardized death rate per 100,000	SMR
University teachers	287	49
Physiotherapists	297	55
Managers in building or contracting	319	54
Local authority senior officers	342	57
Company secretaries and registrars	362	60
Ministers, senior government officials, MPs	371	61
Office managers	377	64
School teachers	396	66
Sales managers	421	70
Architects, town planners	443	74
Civil servants, executive officers	467	78
Postmen	484	81
Medical practitioners	494	81
Coal miners (underground)	822	141
Leather products makers	895	147
Machine tool operators	934	156
Watch repairers	946	154
Coal miners (above ground)	972	160
Steel erectors, riggers	992	164
Fishermen	1028	171
Deck, engineering, officers and pilot's ship	1040	175
Labourers and unskilled workers, all industries	1247	201
Policemen	1270	209
Deck and engine room ratings	1385	233
Bricklayers, labourers	1644	274

Source: Townsend and Davidson (1982), Table 42, p. 194
(NB: SMR refers to the standard mortality rate. Figures in the second column below 100 indicate a below-average mortality rate and those above 100 are above-average rate.)

Mortality rates vary considerably between the regions that make up the United Kingdom. The healthiest part of Britain appears to be the southern belt below a line drawn across the country from the Wash to the Bristol Channel (Table 3 and Figure 5).

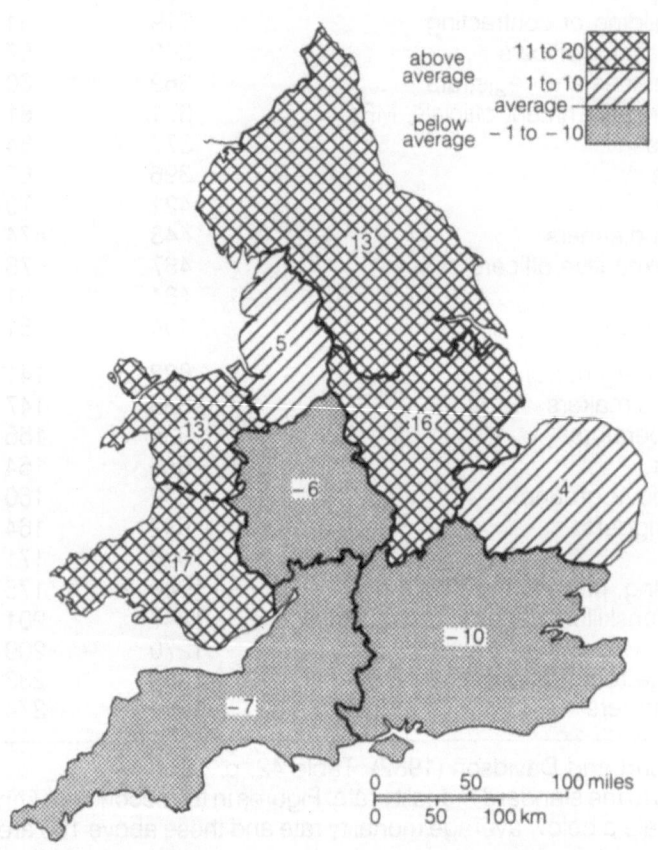

Figure 5 Regional variations in mortality (see explanatory note on Table 3) (Townsend and Davidson, 1982, Table 2, p. 58)

Table 3   Regional variations in mortality

Standard region	SMR age	Standardization age and class
A Northern Yorkshire, Humberside	113	113
B North West	106	105
C East Midlands	116	116
D West Midlands	96	94
E East Anglia	105	104
F South East	90	90
G South West	93	93
H Wales I (south)	114	117
I Wales II (north and west)	110	113
England and Wales	100	100

(When SMR = 100 a plus figure means a higher-than-average mortality and a minus figure a lower-than-average mortality.)

BIRTH WEIGHT AND CLASS

Even when allowance is made for whether it is the first or a subsequent child the poorest occupational class gives birth to three times as many babies under 2500 grams as the richest. About 7 per cent

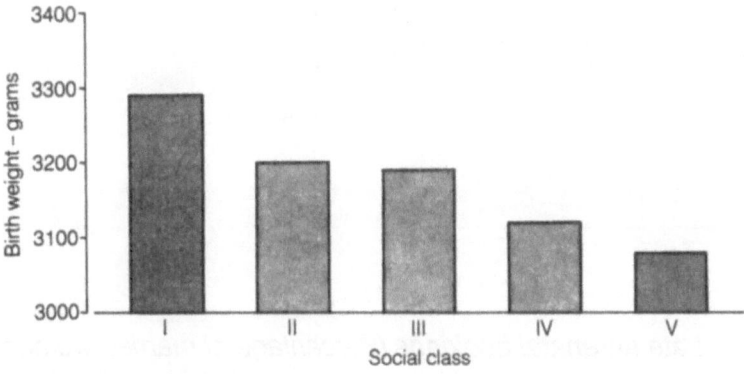

Figure 6 Birth weight averages by social class (primips) (Scotland, 1971–4) (Fenton-Lewis, A. and Modle, W. J. (1982), Health Trends, *1982, 14, 3)*

of all births weigh under 2500 grams. Women in lower social classes give birth to smaller babies. Low birth weight is the best single predictor of perinatal mortality (Figure 6).

HEALTH SERVICE AVAILABILITY AND USAGE BY SOCIAL CLASS

Late antenatal bookings

Late antenatal booking is more frequent in poorer social groups. Late attendance for antenatal care is an effective predictor of subsequent infant morbidity and mortality (Figure 7). Similar class differences have been found in attendance at postnatal examinations, antenatal and postnatal supervision, and uptake of vitamin foods.

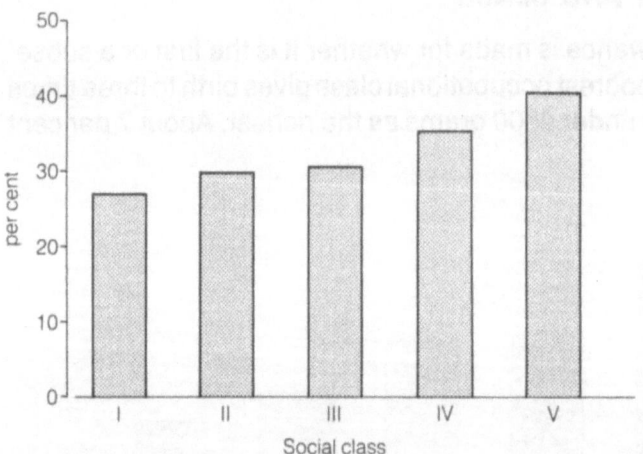

Figure 7 Late antenatal bookings (Percentage of married women in each occupational class making an antenatal booking after more than 20 weeks of gestation, Scotland, 1973) (Brotherston (1976). Data from Scottish Information Services Division. Quoted in Townsend and Davidson (1982), Table 16, p. 82)

Immunization

Uptake of immunization in children is related to social class. Non-uptake is highest in social class V (Figure 8).

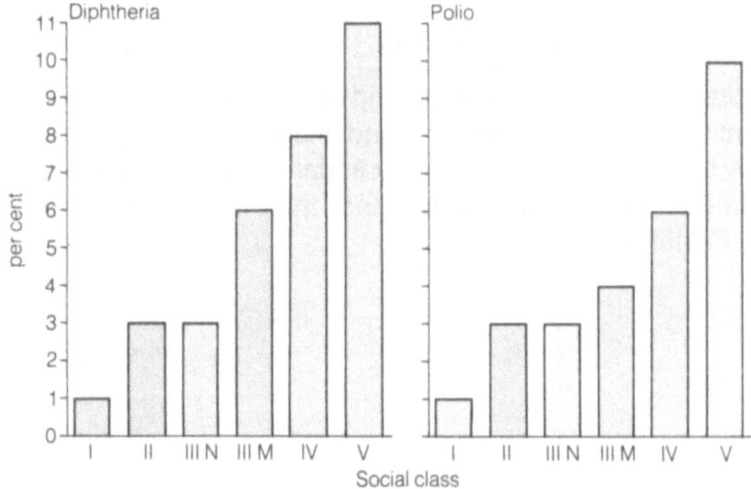

Figure 8 Percentages of children at 7 years not immunized against diphtheria and polio by social class (National Child Development Study (1958 birth cohort). Quoted in Townsend and Davidson (1982), Table 17, p. 83)

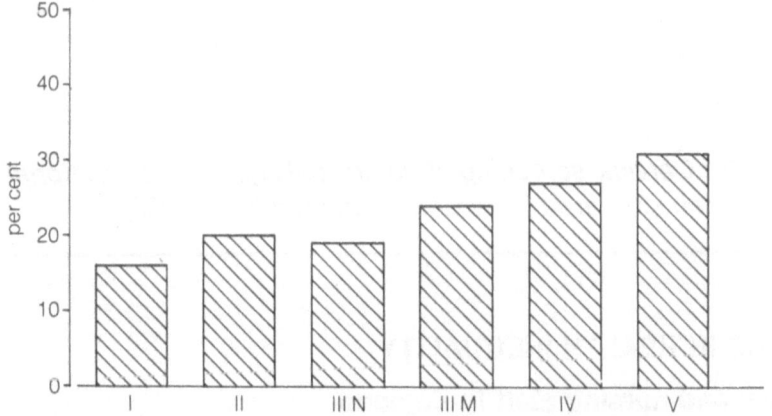

Figure 9 Use of dental services (Percentages of children at 7 who have never visited a dentist) (National Child Development Study (1958 birth cohort). Quoted in Townsend and Davidson (1982), Table 17, p. 83)

Use of dental services

Likewise use of dental services in children is class-related (Figure 9).

Cervical screening by social class

Middle-class women, both married and unmarried, make most use of preventive services. Semi-skilled and unskilled women are much less likely to be screened for cervical cancer even though the death rate from this condition is much higher than in the professional classes (Figure 10).

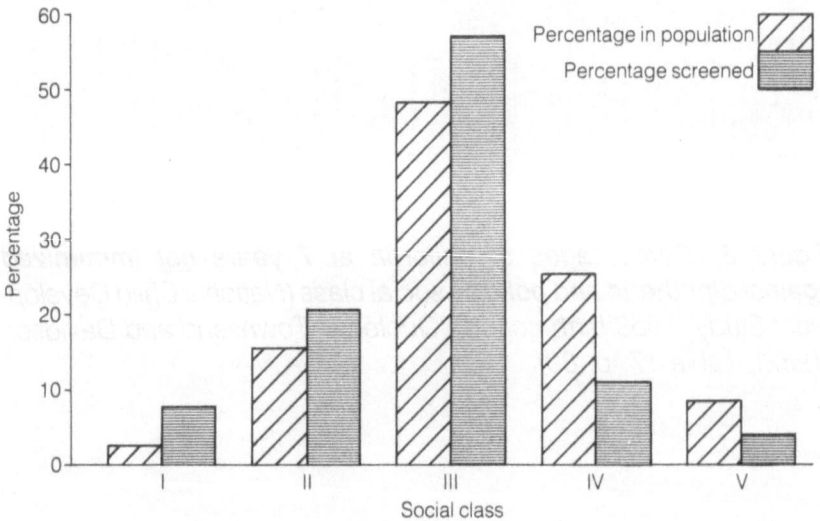

Figure 10 *Cervical screening of women (all ages) by occupational class: Manchester area (Townsend and Davidson, 1982)*

TRENDS IN HEALTH INEQUALITY

Medical and nursing staff in England

The rate of increase in hospital doctors has been nearly seven-fold greater than that in general practitioners (Figure 11a and Table 4). Services outside hospital have been singled out for high priority. In the formative years of the health service two-thirds of the nation's doctors worked in general practice; now two-thirds work in hospital. In absolute terms the increase in numbers of nurses working in hospital has dwarfed the additional numbers working in the community, but the rate of increase has been greater in community nurses (Figure 11b and Table 4).

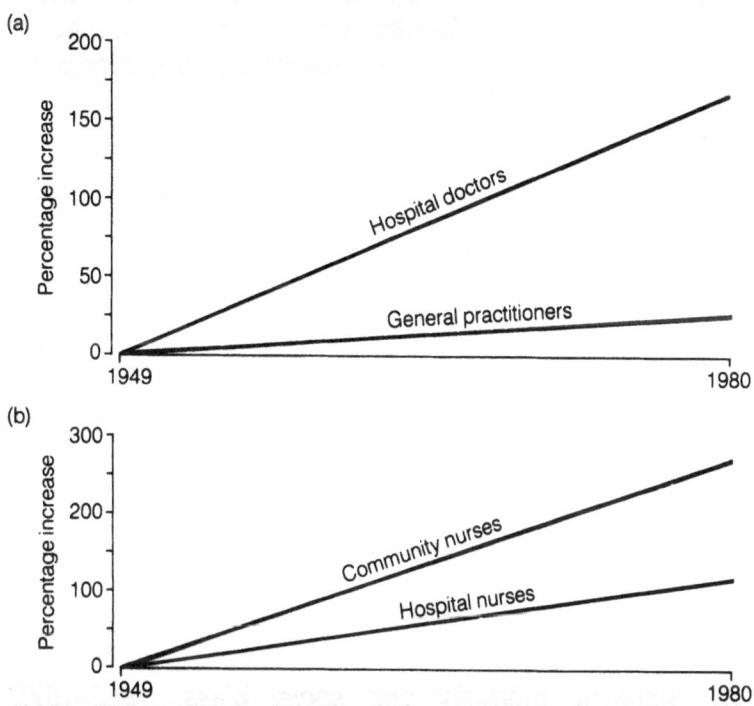

Figure 11 (a) *Medical and* (b) *nursing staff in hospital and general practice, 1949–1980 (Townsend and Davidson (1982), Table C, p. 30)*

Table 4 Medical and nursing staff in hospital and general practice, 1949–1980

Health service personnel		1949	1980
Doctors:	Hospital	11,735	31,421
	General practice	18,000	22,674
Nurses:	Hospital	137,636	297,684
	Community	9529	32,162

Source: Townsend and Davidson (1982)

Maternal deaths

Between 1962 and 1972 the number of mothers dying in childbirth fell by more than one-third. Although the numbers of deaths of wives of professional workers fell less sharply than other classes, inequality between managerial class and manual workers' wives remained about the same. Deaths among women married to unskilled workers were nearly double those of wives of professional workers in 1972 (Figure 12).

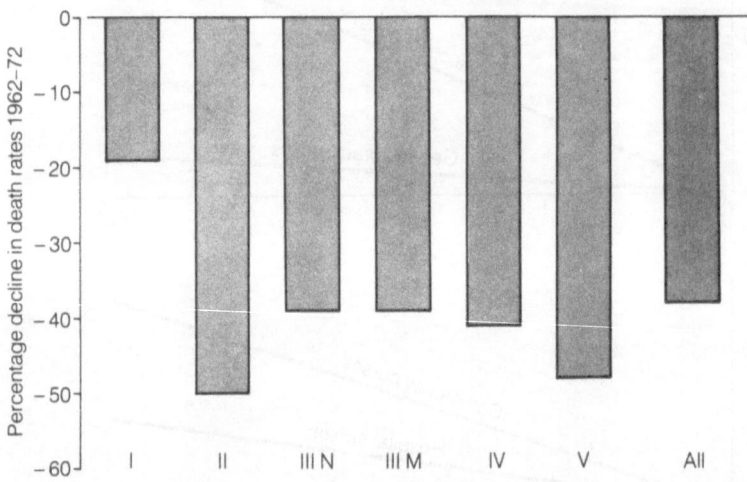

Figure 12 Maternal mortality and social class, 1962–1972 (percentage decline calculated jointly) (Townsend and Davidson, 1982)

Deaths of infants

Between 1950 and 1973 the number of infant deaths fell least in social class V (Figure 13).

Between 1949/1953 and 1959/1963 inequalities between occupational classes I and V in mortality experience widened. By 1970/1972 there was little change in the continuing mortality advantage of class I. Although there was an improvement in the mortality disadvantage of social class V relative to the other social classes, this improvement fell short of restoring the position the class had reached in 1949/1953.

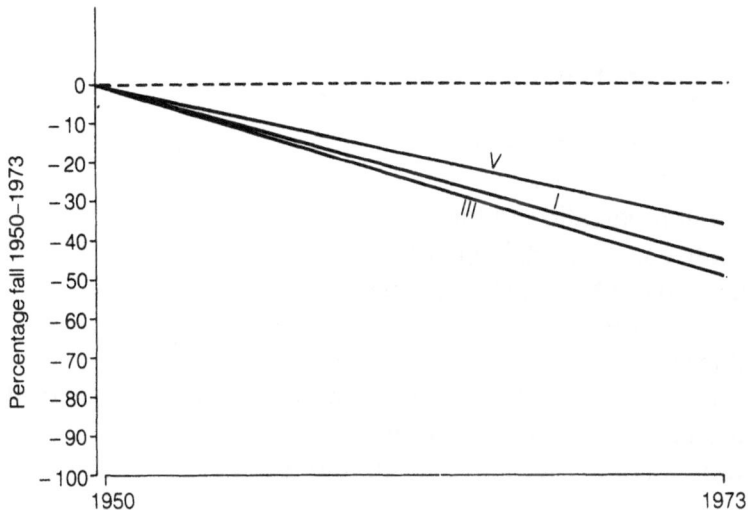

*Figure 13   Deaths of infants in the first week of life, 1950–1973
(Court Report – quoted by Townsend and Davidson (1982), p. 70)*

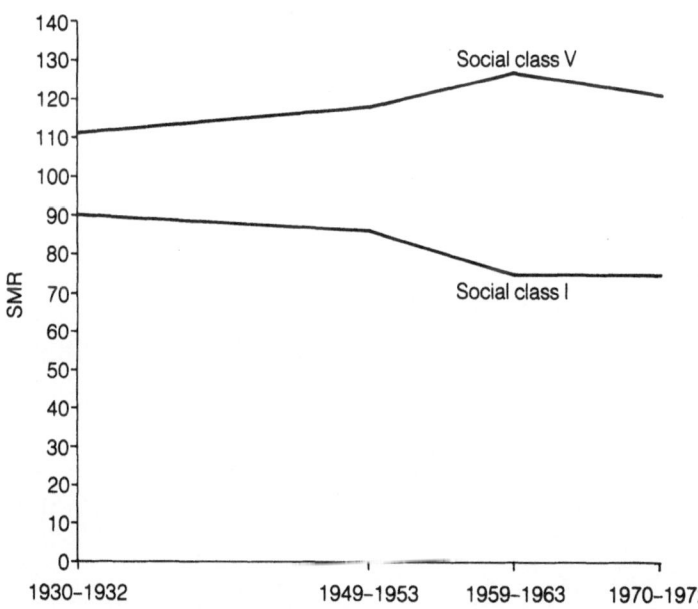

*Figure 14   Mortality of men by occupational class (standard mortality ratios), 1930–1970 (Registrar General. Quoted by Townsend
and Davidson (1982), Table 7, p. 67)*

COMMENT

- Lower classes suffer more from –
  - Accidents
  - Late antenatal bookings
  - Low birth weights
  - Low immunization uptake
  - Lower use of dental services
  - Lower use of cervical cytology
  - Infant mortality
  - All mortality.
- Mortality rates are highest in heavy manual workers and lowest in sedentary non-clerical workers.
- Mortality rates higher in North than in South.

CHAPTER 6

STRUCTURE AND ROLES OF NHS

BASIC LEVELS

In all health care systems there are certain inevitable and essential levels of care and administration (Figure 1). The *levels of care* are:
- self-care
- primary professional care
- general specialist care
- sub-specialist care

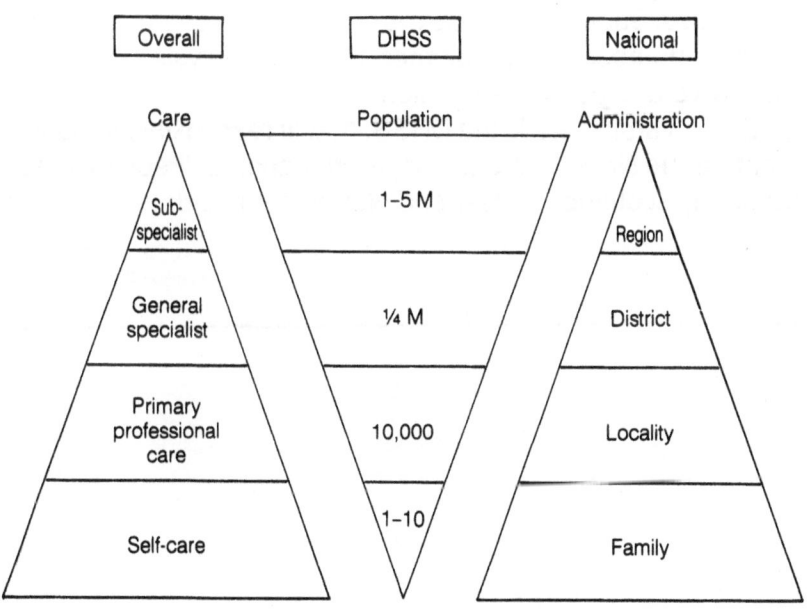

Figure 1   Levels of care—administration

- *Self-care* is where most of medical care takes place. It is where individuals and families care for minor symptoms, self-limiting diseases and for chronic disorders in collaboration with professionals.
- *Primary professional care* – once the decision is taken to consult a professional there are limited choices.

  In the NHS it is the general practitioner who is the portal of entry for most primary care in the NHS, but there is the choice of direct access also to the hospital accident–emergency department and clinics for venereal diseases; nurses in certain places and situations; paramedical services such as clinics for child care, family planning, cervical cytology and breast checks; social services and voluntary disease-organizations; and fringe services such as osteopathy, acupuncture, hypnotherapy and others.
- *General specialist care* is that provided at a district general hospital, with general services for general medicine, general surgery, general OBG, general trauma and orthopaedics, general psychiatry and general paediatrics, plus some other specialties. Sub-specialist care is of specialties such as thoracic surgery, neurosurgery, radiotherapy, renal dialysis and others that serve a region of 1–5 million.
- *DHSS* – overall there is the DHSS, that is responsible to parliament for the NHS. There are separate national directorates for England, Scotland, Wales, and Northern Ireland.

LEVELS OF ADMINISTRATION

Figure 2 shows the numbers of administrative units at each level of care.

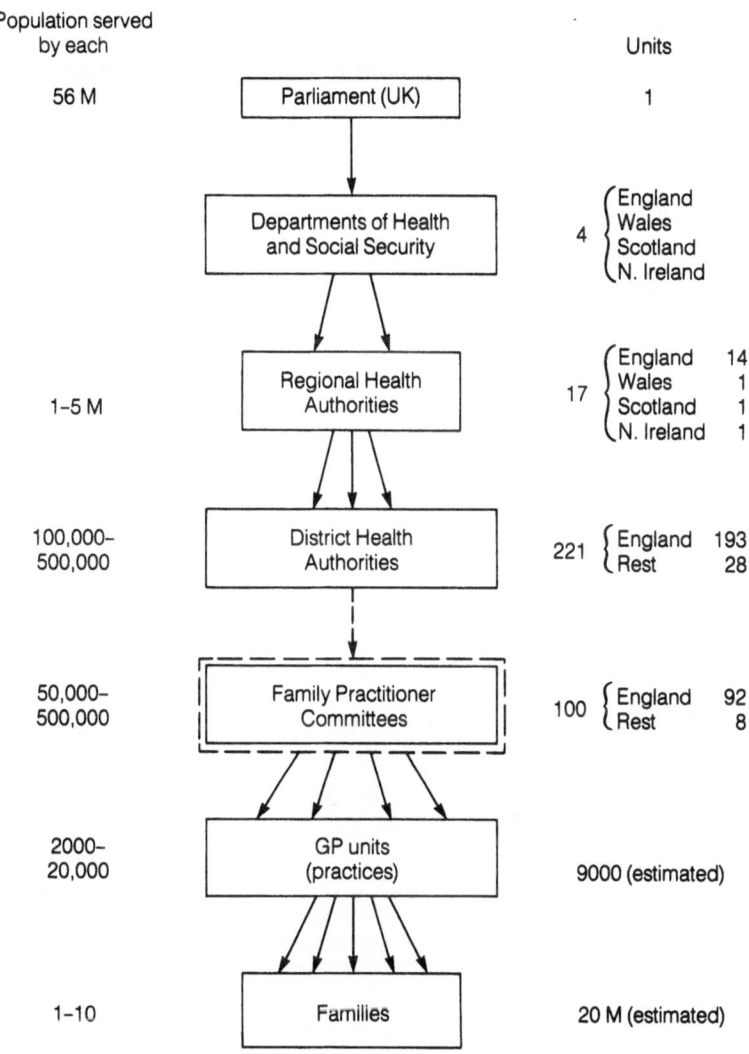

Figure 2   Levels of administration (UK)

COMMENT

- The four *levels of care* in any health systems are:
  - self-care;
  - primary professional care:
  - general specialist care;
  - sub-(super)-specialist care.
- *Each level* has its own population base and administrative structure.
- In the *NHS* the Department of Health and Social Security (DHSS) has overall controls and responsibility.
- The *current problems* within the NHS relate largely to lack of clear and firm control, responsibility and accountability at each level of care and administration.

CHAPTER 7

FACILITIES AND RESOURCES

HOSPITALS

Numbers of hospitals

The number of hospitals in England from 1959 to 1980 is shown in Figure 1 and Table 1. Hospital numbers decreased by 457 (or almost 20 per cent) during this period. Related to the population size the reduction was even greater – 25 per cent.

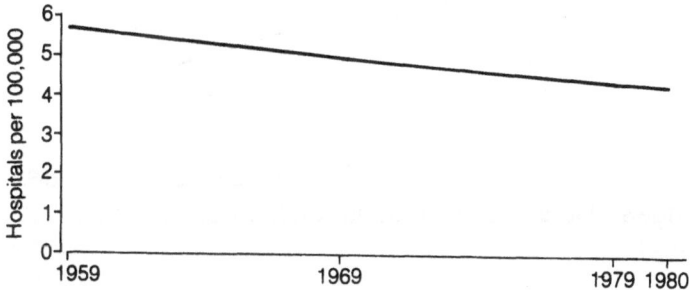

*Figure 1 Hospitals in England, 1959–1980: numbers and rates per 100,000 (*Health and Personal Social Services Statistics, *1982, Table 4.2)*

Table 1 Hospitals in England, 1959–1980: numbers and rates per 100,000

	1959	1969	1979	1980	*Percentage change 1959–1980*
Population of England (million)	43	46	46.4	46.4	—
Number of hospitals	2441	2293	2023	1984	–19
Hospitals per 100,000	5.7	5.0	4.4	4.3	–25

Source: *Health and Personal Social Services Statistics*, 1982, Table 4.2

Bed size

National policies (Figure 2 and Table 2) have resulted in reductions in small (under 250 beds) and huge (over 1000 beds) hospitals, maintenance of numbers of hospitals of 250–500 beds, and increase in numbers of those with 500–1000 beds.

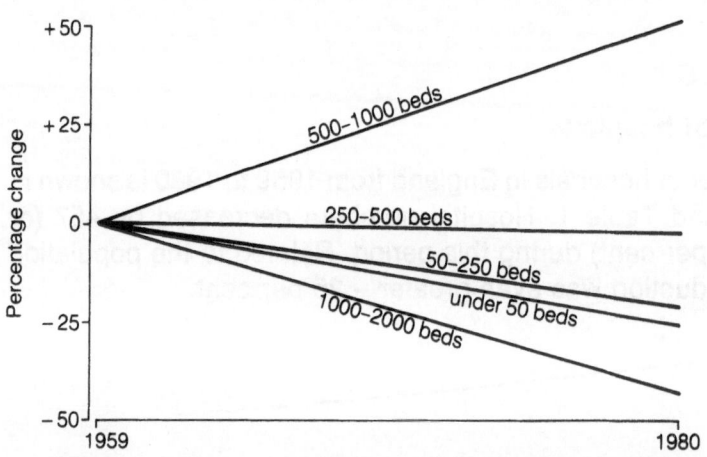

Figure 2 Hospitals in England, 1959–1980: bed size and percentage changes (Health and Personal Social Services Statistics, 1982, Table 4.2)

Table 2 Hospitals in England, 1959–1980: bed size and percentage changes

Bed size of hospital	1959	1969	1979	1980	Percentage change 1959–1980
Under 50	977	825	742	727	− 26
50–250	1011	991	819	802	− 21
250–500	243	254	243	239	− 2
500–1000	119	149	178	180	+ 52
1000–2000	63	65	41	36	− 43
over 2000	28	9	0	0	—
All hospitals	2441	2293	2023	1984	− 19

Source: *Health and Personal Social Services Statistics*, 1982, Table 4.2

Non-psychiatric and psychiatric hospitals

Different trends occurred in non-psychiatric and psychiatric hospitals. The numbers of *non-psychiatric hospitals* of up to 500 beds

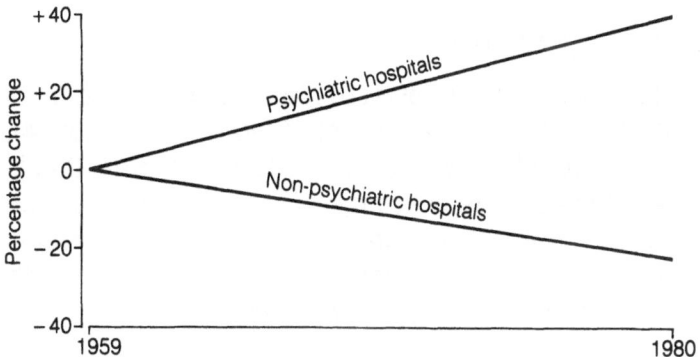

Figure 3   Hospitals in England, 1959–1980: non-psychiatric and psychiatric – bed size and percentage changes (Health and Personal Social Services Statistics, *1982, Table 4.2)*

Table 3 Hospitals in England, 1959–1980: non-psychiatric and psychiatric – bed size and percentage changes

Bed size	1959	1969	1979	1980	Percentage change 1959–1980
Non-psychiatric hospitals					
Under 50 beds	912	755	601	575	– 37
50–250	925	896	705	690	– 36
250–500	216	220	190	180	– 17
500–1000	76	87	103	105	+ 47
Over 1000	9	6	10	10	+ 11
All	2138	1964	1609	1560	– 22
Psychiatric hospitals					
Under 50 beds	65	70	141	152	+ 134
50–250	86	95	114	112	+ 30
250–500	27	34	53	59	+ 119
500–1000	43	62	75	75	+ 74
Over 1000	82	68	31	26	– 315
All	303	329	414	424	+ 40

Source: *Health and Personal Social Services Statistics*, 1982, Table 4.2

fell but there were increases in hospitals with over 500 beds. The opposite trends occurred in *psychiatric hospitals*: falls in those over 1000 beds and increases in those under 1000 beds (Figure 3 and Table 3).

Allocated and occupied beds

Another way of measuring hospital resources is by the numbers of beds allocated per 1000 of the population (Figure 4 and Table 4), and of the beds occupied. This gives the *occupancy rates*, that is the percentages of hospital beds occupied. From 1959 to 1980 the rates fell from 86 per cent to 80 per cent. Probably the chief reason why the occupancy rates have fallen is because district health authorities do not have funds to staff hospitals.

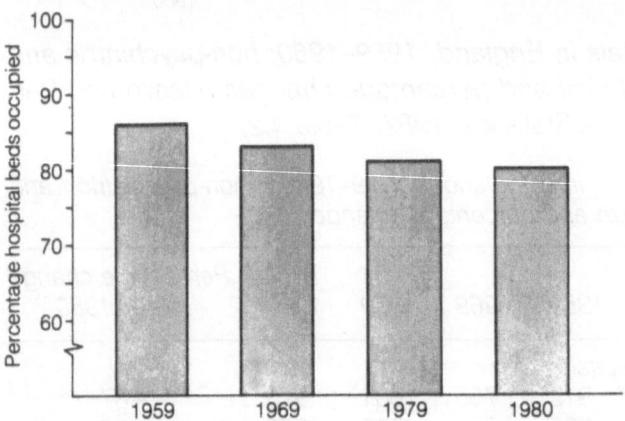

Figure 4   Hospital bed occupancy rates (England, 1959–1980) (Health and Personal Social Services Statistics, *1982, Table 4.6)*

Table 4   Allocated and occupied hospital beds per 1000 (England, 1959– 1980) and occupancy rates

	1959	1969	1979	1980
Allocated beds	10.6	9.5	7.8	7.7
Occupied beds	9.1	7.8	6.3	6.2
Occupancy rates (%)	86	83	81	80

Source: *Health and Personal Social Services Statistics*, 1982, Table 4.6

The distributions of *occupied beds* of *non-psychiatric and psychiatric hospitals* (Figure 5 and Table 5) are shown in rates per 1000 of the population. There were reductions in all categories, but greatest in the psychiatric beds occupied. Thus in relation to the population served, fewer hospital beds were occupied but, as shown in Chapter 10, there were more persons admitted, suggesting greater efficiency.

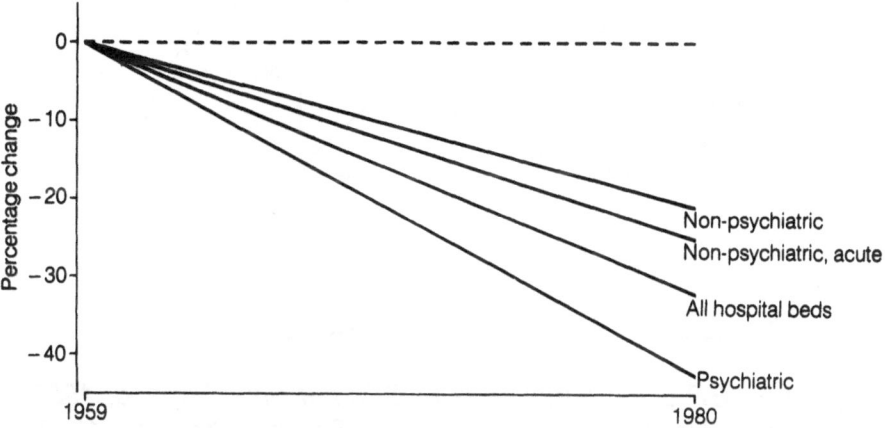

Figure 5 Hospital beds (England, 1959–1980): beds occupied per 1000, and percentage changes (Health and Personal Social Services Statistics, *1982, from Table 4.6)*

Table 5 Hospital beds (England, 1959–1980): beds occupied per 1000, and percentage change

	1959	1969	1979	1980	Percentage change 1959–1980
Non-psychiatric	4.7	4.2	3.7	3.7	− 21
(Non-psychiatric-acute)	(3.5)	(3.1)	(2.6)	(2.6)	(− 25)
Psychiatric	4.4	3.6	2.6	2.5	− 43
All occupied beds	9.1	7.8	6.3	6.2	− 32

Source: *Health and Personal Social Services Statistics*, 1982, from Table 4.6

GENERAL PRACTICE UNITS

The organization of NHS general practice has changed considerably. The moves towards group practice have been considerable (Figure 6 and Table 6). This has led to fewer GP units (Figure 7 and Table 7). Thus with more GPs working together from central premises the numbers of such units have continued to decrease.

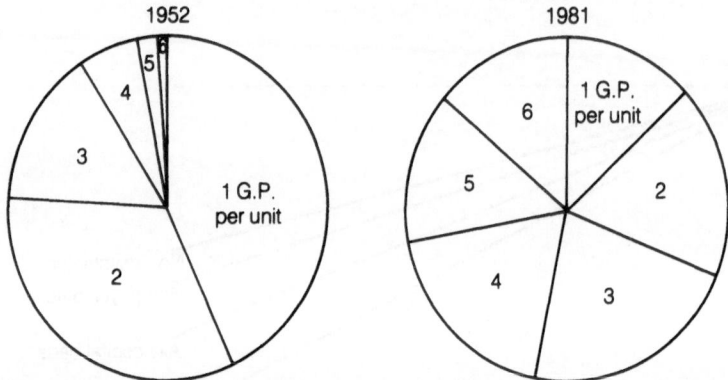

Figure 6   GP units: percentage of GPs per unit (England, 1952 and 1981) (Health and Personal Social Services Statistics, *1982, Table 3.22)*

Table 6   GP units: percentages of GPs per unit (England, 1952 and 1981)

Size of GP unit (numbers of GPs per unit)	Percentage GPs	
	1952	1981
× 1	43	13
× 2	33	18
× 3	15	22
× 4	6	19
× 5	2	14
× 6 or more	1	14
Total (%)	100	100

Source: *Health and Personal Social Services Statistics,* 1982, Table 3.22

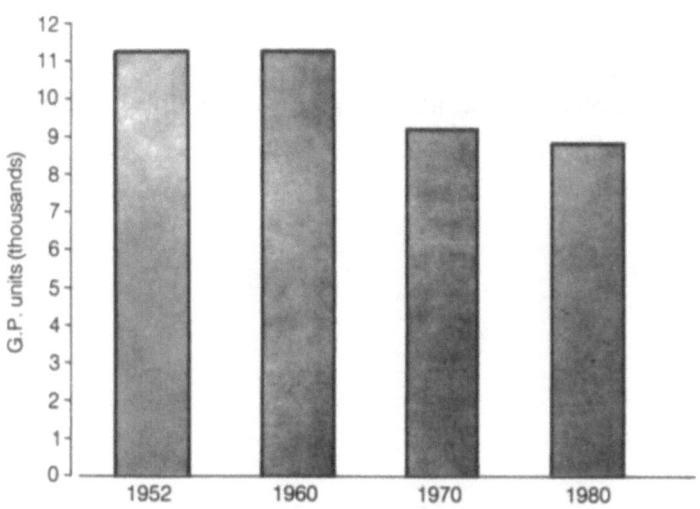

Figure 7 GP units (England and Wales) and principals (1952–1980) (Health and Personal Social Services Statistics, *1982, Table 3.22 and provisional data from DHSS)*

Table 7 GP units (England and Wales) and principals (1952–1980)

Numbers of GPs per unit	1952	1960	1970	1980	Percentage change 1952–1980
×1	7400	5975	4034	3089	−58
×2	2838	3481	2353	2008	−29
×3	860	1394	1623	1704	+98
×4	258	448	750	1052	+308
×5	69	119	290	553	+701
×6+	32	66	173	430	+1244
Total number of units	11,457	11,483	9223	8336	−24
GP principals in England and Wales	17,204	19,915	20,357	23,184	+35

Source: *Health and Personal Social Services Statistics,* 1982, Table 3.22 and provisional data from DHSS

CHEMISTS AND DRUG STORES

The numbers of these facilities are declining, with fewer of the smaller units and more of the larger units (Figure 8) (1974–1980 showed a decline of 8 per cent).

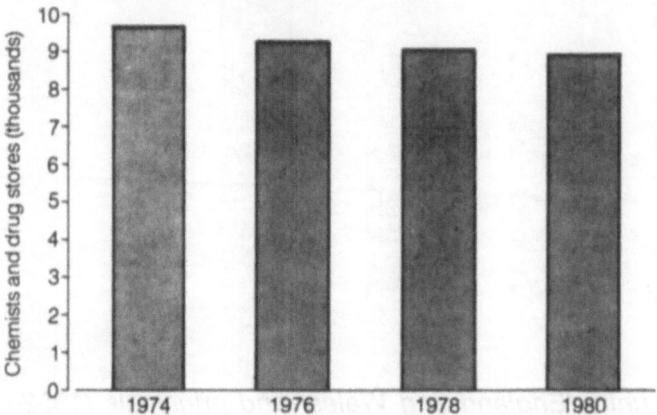

*Figure 8   Number of chemists and drug store units (England, 1974–1980) (*Health and Personal Social Services Statistics, *1982, Table 5.7)*

COMMUNITY HOMES

Homes provided by local authorities

The numbers of such welfare homes have more than doubled since 1959 (Figure 9 and Table 8). Most have between 30 and 70 beds (Figure 10 and Table 9).

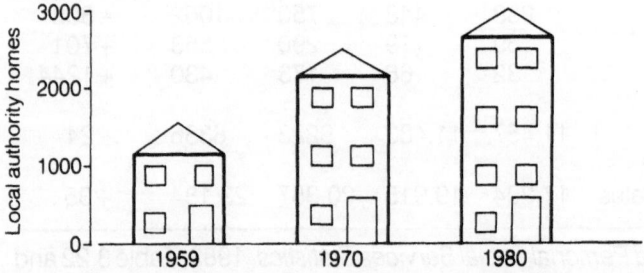

*Figure 9   Local authority homes, England, 1959–1980 (*Health and Personal Social Services Statistics, *1982, Table 7.1)*

Table 8   Local authority homes, England, 1959–1980

	1959	1970	1980
Numbers of homes	1140	2166	2658
Places (for persons)	77,000	92,880	126,000

Source: *Health and Personal Social Services Statistics*, 1982, Table 7.1)

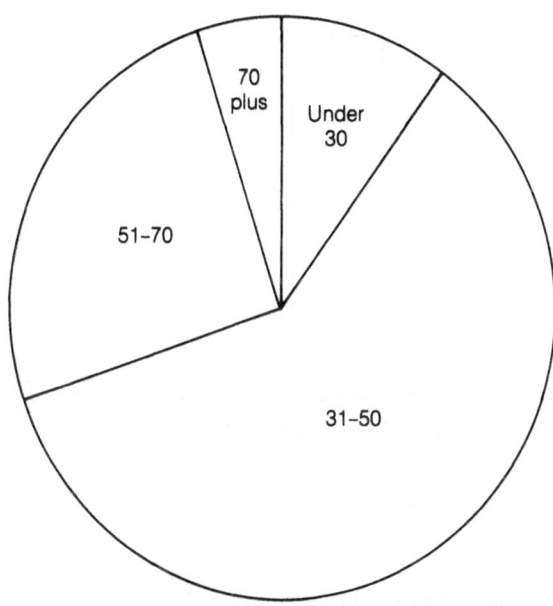

Figure 10   Size of local authority homes (places per home) (Health and Personal Social Services Statistics, *1982, Table 7.2)*

Table 9   Size of local authority homes (places per home)

	Places per home				
	under 30	31–50	51–70	71–150	151+
Percentage	10	60	25	5	Less than 1

Source: *Health and Personal Social Services Statistics*, 1982, Table 7.2

Private and voluntary homes

The numbers of these homes, and the places that they offer, have increased also; Figure 11 and Table 10 show the trends.

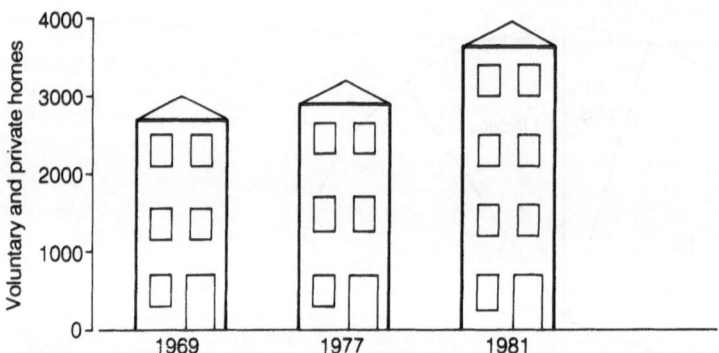

Figure 11   Voluntary and private homes, England, 1969–1981
(Health and Personal Social Services Statistics, *1982, Table 7.3)*

Table 10   Voluntary and private homes, England, 1969–1981

	1969	1977	1981
Voluntary homes			
Numbers	992	1038	1118
Places	31,582	33,222	36,810
Private homes			
Numbers	1706	1861	2515
Places	21,741	28,000	39,300
Total			
Numbers	2698	2899	3628
Places	53,323	61,222	72,110

Source: *Health and Personal Social Services Statistics*, 1982, Table 7.3

Hostels and homes for mentally ill and handicapped

The numbers of hostels and homes for the mentally ill and handicapped show much larger increases in local authority units than in the voluntary and private units (Figure 12 and Table 11).

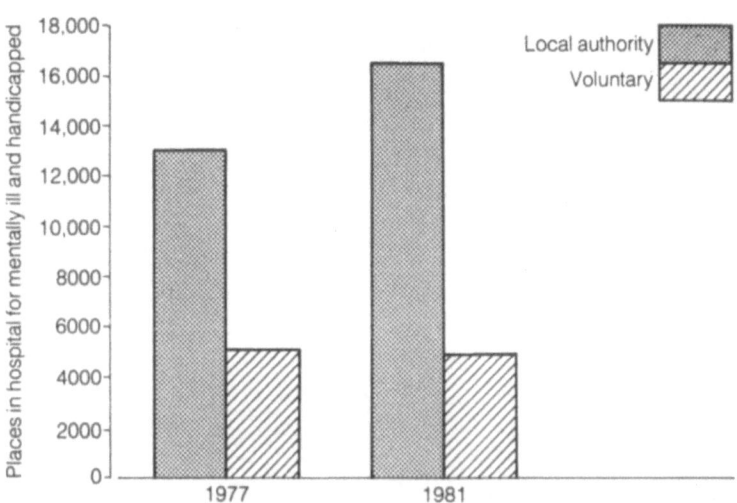

*Figure 12   Homes and hostels for mentally ill and handicapped, England, 1977–1981 (*Health and Personal Social Services Statistics, 1982, Table 7.4)

Table 11   Homes and hostels for mentally ill and handicapped, England, 1977–1981

	1977	1981
Local authority		
Hostels/homes	879	1340
Places	12,940	16,750
Voluntary		
Hostels/homes	248	297
Places	5130	5044

Source: *Health and Personal Social Services Statistics*, 1982, Table 7.4

PRIVATE MEDICAL SERVICES

NHS private beds

Although the numbers of private pay beds in NHS have been greatly reduced (Figure 13 and Table 12), the numbers of persons treated per bed have almost doubled because of shorter stay.

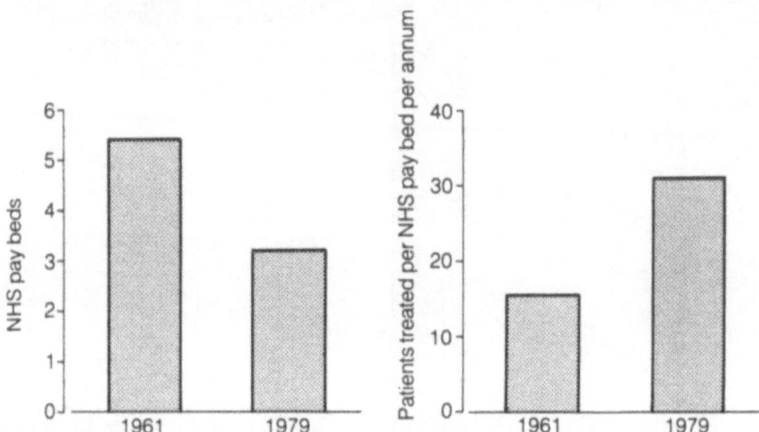

Figure 13 NHS pay beds – numbers allocated and persons treated per bed (Social Trends, 1983, Table 7.25)

Table 12 NHS pay beds – numbers allocated and persons treated per bed

	1961	1980
Pay NHS beds allocated (in thousands)	5.4	3.2
Patients treated per bed per annum	15.4	31.0

Source: *Social Trends*, 1983, Table 7.25

Private hospitals

The numbers of private hospitals and nursing homes have increased and more persons are insured under provident schemes for medical care (Figure 14). However:

● only 7 per cent of the population are so insured;
● only 6 per cent of all hospital beds are in private hosptals;
● only 2 per cent of all acute beds are in private hospitals.

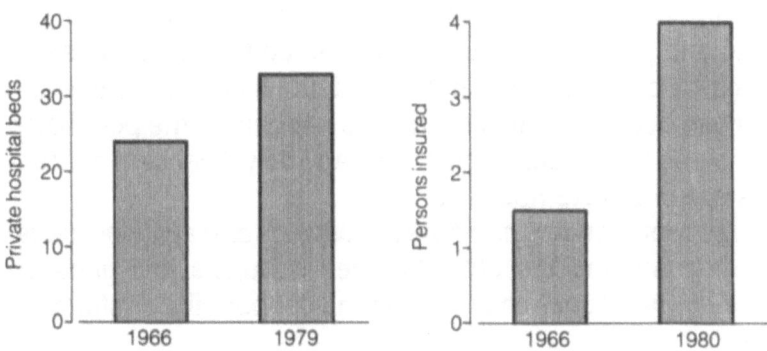

Figure 14 Private hospital beds and numbers insured under private medical schemes (Social Trends, 1983, Chart 7.26)

COMMENT

- The number of *NHS hospitals* decreased by one-quarter from 1959 to 1980 related to population size.
- Available *occupied hospital beds* were reduced by 32 per cent.
- Changes in *hospital bed-size* have reflected political policies. There has been an increase of 52 per cent in hospitals of 500–1000 beds and marked decreases in small hospitals of less than 250 beds (by 25 per cent) and in large hospitals of over 1000 beds (by almost 50 per cent).
- *Occupancy* of available hospital beds was 80 per cent in 1980 compared with 86 per cent in 1959.
- In *general practice* there has been a major trend to larger partnership groups. In 1952, 76 per cent of GPs were in solo and two-man practices; in 1981 it was 31 per cent. In 1981, 28 per cent of GPs were in groups of five or more doctors.
- The number of *GP principals* increased by 35 per cent from 1952 to 1980.
- The number of *general practice units* (practices) declined by 24 per cent (1952–1980) because of larger partnerships.
- The number of *chemist and drug stores* is decreasing, the smaller ones are being replaced by larger stores.

- *Community residential and nursing homes* are increasing in public and private sectors but still are too few to meet needs.
- *Private medical care* has increased both in NHS hospitals and in private hospitals, but less than 10 per cent of the population are insured for private medical care and only 2 per cent of acute beds are in private hospitals.
- The policy of reducing *numbers of hospitals and available beds*, and of promoting the 500–1000-bed hospitals has gone on apace but has not been evaluated in cost-benefits or effectiveness.
- The trend in *general practice* towards larger groups in fewer units has been encouraged by NHS financial inducements but there has been no evaluation of quality benefits.
- Major *changes in policies* in health care have taken place without any built-in reliable evaluation.

CHAPTER 8

PERSONNEL IN NHS

ALL NHS STAFF

The National Health Service (NHS) is one of the largest employers in the United Kingdom. There are more than 1 million persons directly employed by the NHS (Figure 1 and Table 1).

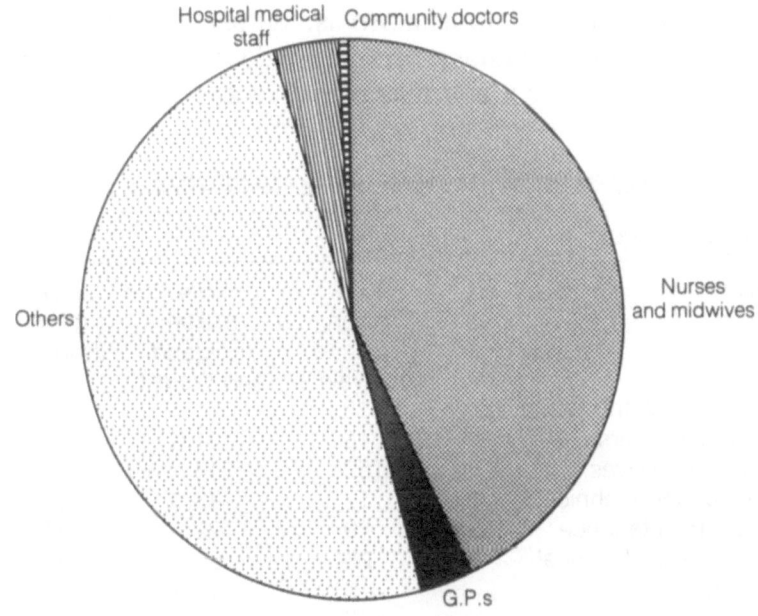

Figure 1   Personnel employed by NHS in the UK in 1981 (numbers rounded off) (Personal data from DHSS and other health departments)

Whole-time equivalents	Hospital doctors and dentists	Doctors in community medicine	Nurses and midwives	General prac-titioners	Others	Total
England	34,600	4400	396,000	23,740	391,260	850,000
Wales	2000	300	24,400	1500	26,800	55,000
Scotland	5300	800	58,600	3300	56,000	124,000
N. Ireland	1500	200	17,300	800	14,600	37,400
Totals	43,400	5700	476,300	29,240	554,640	1,066,400
Percentages	4	0.5	43	3	49.5	100

Source: Personal data from DHSS and other health departments

Types of NHS staff employed (WTEs)

The types of staff expressed as whole-time equivalents (WTEs) for England and Wales in 1949 and 1974, and for England in 1981 (Table 2) show that the breakdown is: nurses and midwives; ancillary staff (such as laundry, catering, orderlies, porters, domestics, telephonists, etc.); and administrative and clerical staff –

Table 2 NHS staff directly employed in WTEs: 1949, 1974 and 1981

Numbers (thousands)	1949	1974	1981
Population	43.8 million (England and Wales)	46.4 million (England and Wales)	47 million (England)
Hospital medical and dental staff	12	31.5	39
General practitioners	15	21.5	23.7
Nurses and midwives	150	314	396
Professional and technical	14	43.6	67.1
Works and maintenance	19	22	27
Administrative and clerical	25	83	108
Ambulance	9	17.5	18.3
Ancillary	158	163.4	167
Total NHS staff	400	675	826

Source: Health and Personal Social Services Statistics, 1982, Table 3.1, and personal data from DHSS

those are the largest categories. Table 2 also shows that the number more than doubled from 1949 to 1981 for a population increase of under 8 per cent.

Types of NHS staff employed in rates per 1000 of population

Figure 2 and Table 3 show the rates in 1949, 1974 and 1981. These demonstrate the rates of increase for each group. The major increases occurred in professional and technical staff, in administrators and clerks, hospital medical staff and nurses and midwives. Note the less than average rise in general practitioners.

Table 3 NHS employed staff, in rates per 1000 of population, 1949, 1974 and 1981

Whole-time equivalents	1949	1974	1981	Proportionate change 1949–1981
All NHS staff	91.3	145.5	175.7	×1.92
Hospital medical and dental	2.7	6.8	8.4	×3.1
GPs	3.4	4.9	5.0	×1.5
Nurses and midwives	34.3	67.7	84.3	×2.46
Professional and technical	3.2	9.4	14.3	×4.46
Works and maintenance	4.3	4.7	5.7	×1.33
Administrative and clerical	5.7	17.8	23.0	×4.04
Ambulance	2.1	3.6	3.9	×1.85
Ancillary	36.0	35.2	35.5	×0.99
Population	43.8 million (England and Wales)	46.4 million (England and Wales)	47 million (England)	×1.07

Source: Health and Personal Social Services Statistics, 1982, Table 3.1 and other personal data from DHSS)

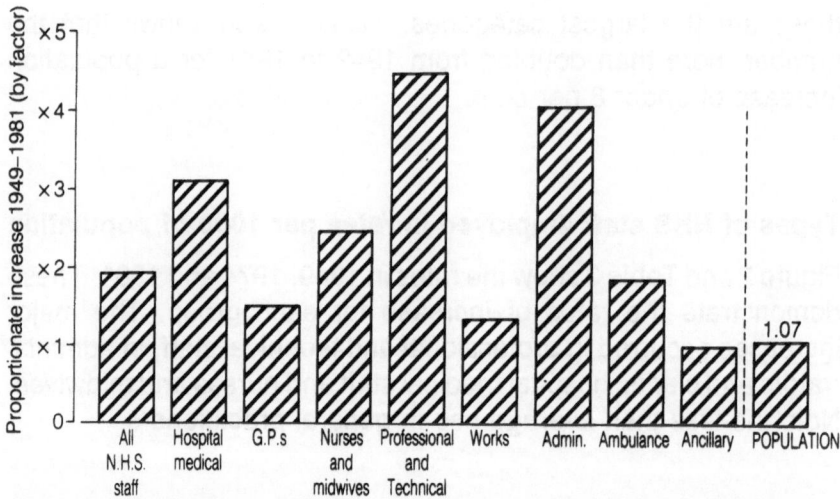

*Figure 2   NHS staff employed, in rates per 1000 of population, 1949–1981 (*Health and Personal Social Services Statistics, *1982, Table 3.1, and personal data from DHSS)*

HOSPITAL MEDICAL STAFF

The numbers of hospital consultants and junior hospital doctors (Figure 3 and Table 4) show that the increases in consultants

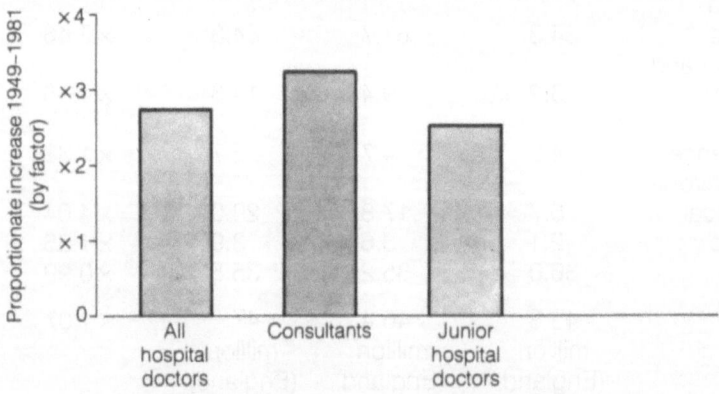

*Figure 3   Numbers (WTE) of hospital doctors, 1949–1981 (*Health and Personal Social Services Statistics, *1982, Table 3.4, and other personal data from DHSS)*

(×3.25) from 1949 to 1981 were greater than for junior hospital doctors (×2.52). These are WTE numbers unrelated to population size. (Note that in rates per 1000 population, in Figure 3 and Table 4, the increases were greater.)

Table 4   Numbers (WTE) of hospital doctors, 1949–1981

WTE	1949 (England and Wales)	1965 (England and Wales)	1981 (England)	Porportionate change 1949–1981
Consultants	3488	6912	11,347	×3.25
Junior hospital doctors	8247	11,993	20,795	×2.52
All hospital doctors	11,735	18,905	32,142	×2.74

Source: *Health and Personal Social Services Statistics*, 1982, Table 3.4, and other personal data from DHSS

Sex distribution

The sex distributions of hospital doctors (Figure 4 and Table 5) show that among junior hospital doctors there are twice as many females as among consultants. This shows the beginning of the effects of more equal numbers of males and females coming out of medical schools.

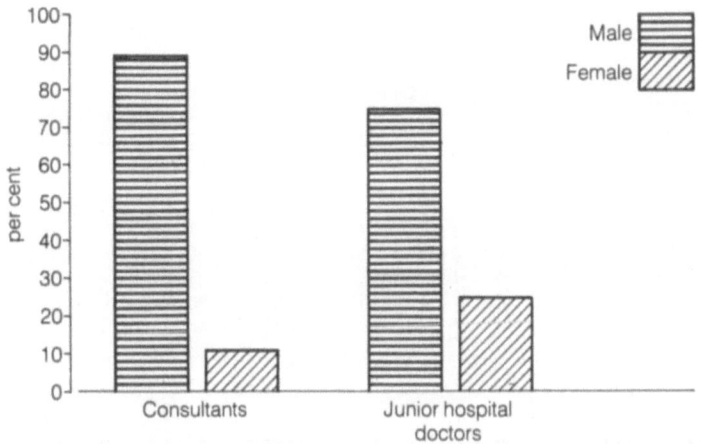

Figure 4   Sex distributions of hospital doctors in England, 1981 (Health and Personal Social Services Statistics, *1982, Table 3.4*)

Table 5   Sex distribution of hospital doctors in England, 1981

	Consultants	Junior hospital doctors	All
Male (%)	89	75	80
Female (%)	11	25	20
Numbers (WTE)	(11,347)	(20,793)	(32,142)

Source: *Health and Personal Social Services Statistics*, 1982, Table 3.4

The hospital specialties

Figure 5 and Table 6 show the largest specialties with more than 100 consultants (WTE). The largest definable groups of specialties are:

- anaesthetics (1528.2)
- psychiatry (1368.8)
- pathology (1082.2)

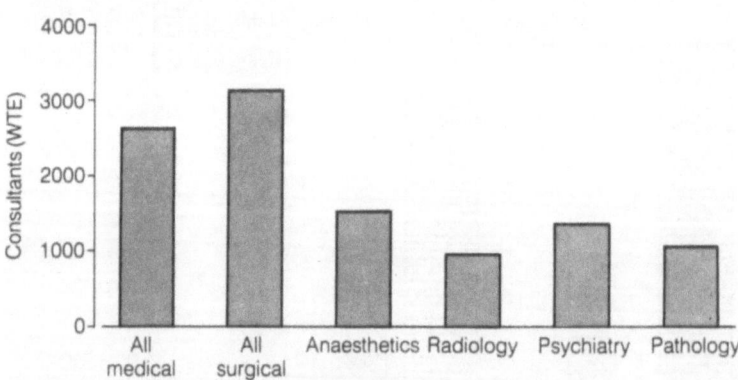

Figure 5   Hospital specialties: numbers (WTE) of consultants in main specialties (England, 1981) (Health and Personal Social Services Statistics, *1982, Table 3.8*)

Table 6   Hospital specialties: numbers (WTE) of consultants in main specialties (England, 1981)

Specialty	Numbers (WTE)
Medical	
General medical	886.2
Rheumatism/rehabilitation	198.2
Diseases of chest	175.1
Dermatology	180.2
Cardiology	101.5
Genito-urinary medicine	101.4
Geriatric	391.4
Neurology	138.5
Paediatrics	447.9
All medical	2620.4
Surgical	
General surgery	836.1
Ear, nose and throat	336.8
Ophthalmology	300.5
Trauma and orthopaedics	597.7
Accident–emergency	121.3
Urology	140.6
Cardiothoracic	104.4
Obstetrics–gynaecology	626.5
All Surgical	3113.9
Anaesthetics	1528.5
Radiotherapy	179.8
Radiology	774.4
Psychiatry	1368.8
Pathology	1082.2
All consultants	11,347.0

Source: *Health and Personal Social Services Statistics*, 1982, Table 3.8

Place of birth

In 1981 just over two-thirds of hospital doctors were born in the United Kingdom and Irish Republic (Figure 6 and Table 7). The proportions in various grades show difference. The proportions of those born 'elsewhere' are lowest in consultant and pre-registration posts.

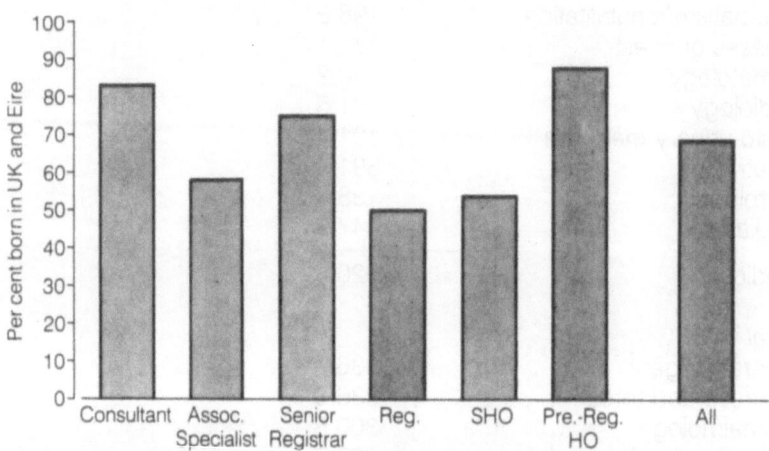

Figure 6   Place of birth of hospital doctors in grades, England, 1981 (percentages) (Hospital and Personal Social Services Statistics, 1982, Table 3.10)

Table 7   Place of birth of hospital doctors in grades, England, 1981 (percentages)

	Consultant	Associate specialists	Senior registrar	Registrar	Senior house officer (SHO)	Pre-registration HO	All
Born in UK and Eire	83	58	75	50	54	88	69
Born elsewhere	17	42	25	50	46	12	31

GENERAL PRACTITIONERS

Numbers of general practitioners

The numbers of general practitioners in the NHS in Figure 7 and Table 8 show steady increases in principals and trainees, and a fall in assistants.

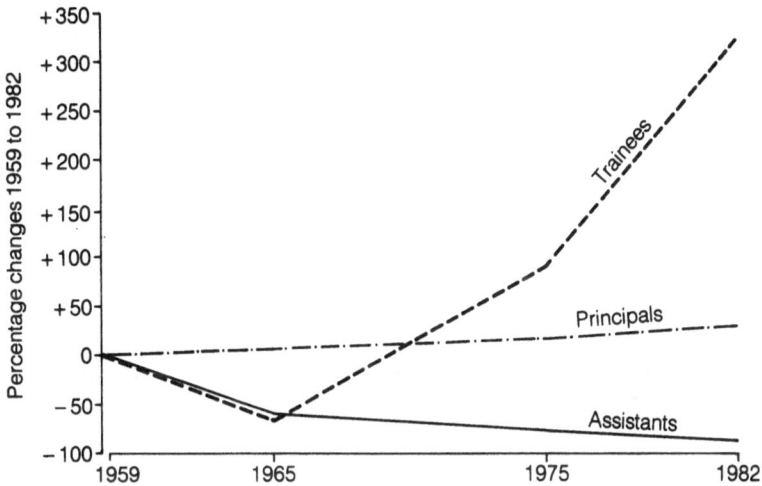

Figure 7 Numbers of GPs in NHS, 1955–1983, percentage changes (Personal data from DHSS)

Table 8   Numbers of GPs in NHS, 1955–1983

	1959	1965	1975	1982 (estimated)
Principals	21,150	22,400	24,644	27,500
Assistants	1800	820	441	250
Trainees	450	154	882	1900
Totals	23,400	23,374	25,967	29,650

Source: Personal data from DHSS

Persons per GP

Over 95 per cent of the public are registered with a general practitioner in the NHS. With increasing numbers of GPs and a fairly static population the numbers of persons per GP principal have been decreasing (Figure 8 and Table 9).

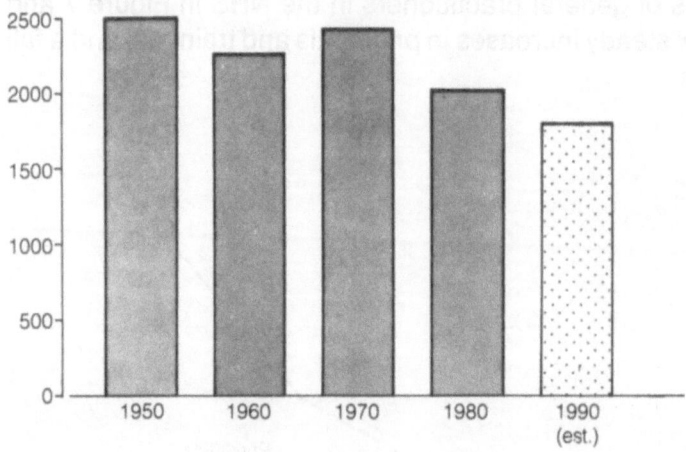

Figure 8   Numbers of persons per NHS GP, 1950–1990 (Personal data from DHSS)

Table 9   Numbers of persons per NHS GP, 1950–1990

	1950	1960	1970	1980	1990 (estimated)
Persons per NHS GP Principal	2500	2257	2413	2017	1800

Source: Personal data from DHSS

National trends

The mean numbers of persons per NHS GP have gone down in England and Wales and Scotland but have gone up in Northern Ireland (Figure 9).

The GP profiles

The GP profiles (Figure 10a–c and Table 10a–c) show their age distribution, sex distribution and place of birth.

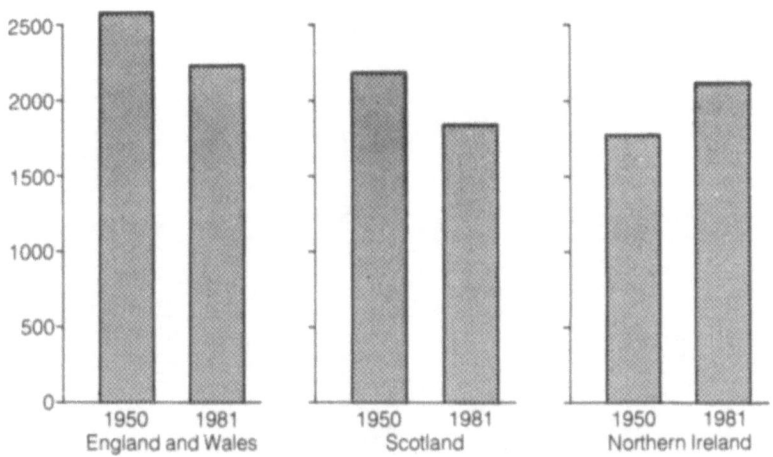

Figure 9   Numbers of persons per GP, 1950 and 1981, in England and Wales, Scotland and Northern Ireland (Personal data from DHSS)

Table 10a   Age distribution of GPs, 1970 (percentages)

Under 30	30–	40–	50–	60–	70+
2	30	30	25	10	3

Table 10b   Sex distribution of GPs (percentages)

	1970	1980
Male	90	83
Female	10	17

Table 10c   Place of birth of GPs (percentages)

	1970	1980
Born in UK and Eire	86	81
Born elsewhere	14	19

Source: *Health and Personal Social Services Statistics*, 1982, Table 3.23 and 3.24

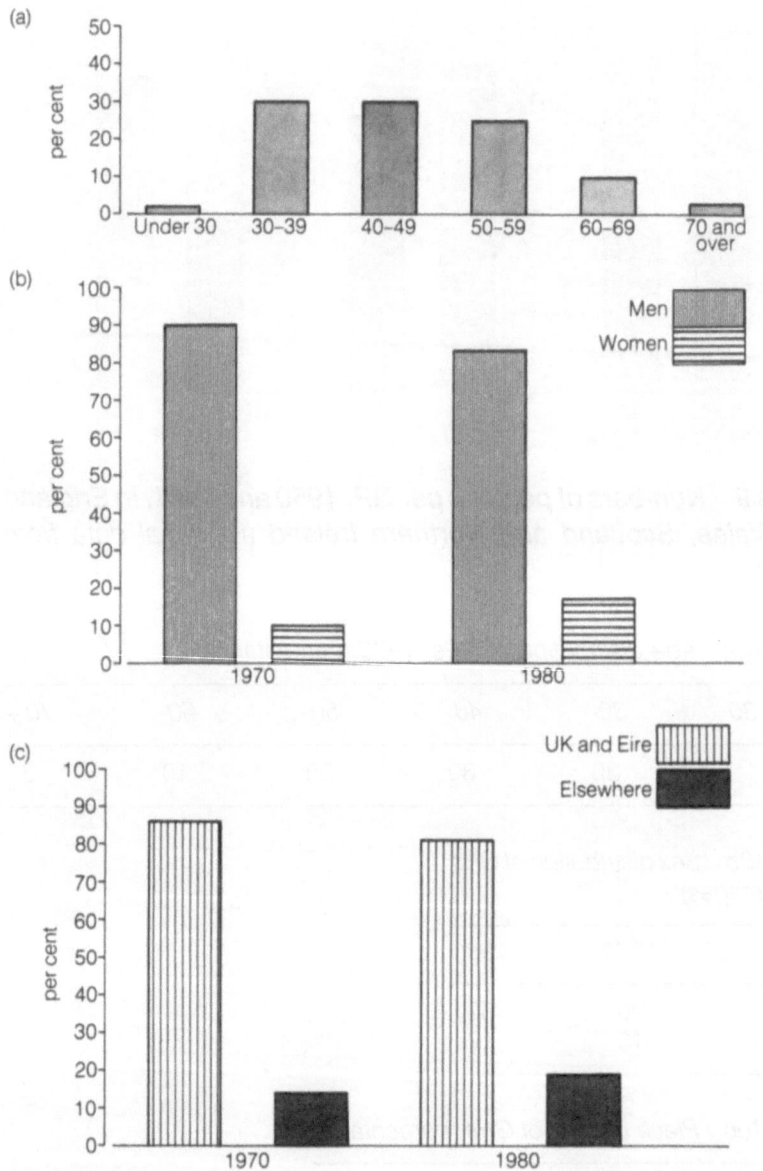

Figure 10   GPs in NHS – distribution (1970 and 1980): (a) Age; (b) sex; (c) place of birth (Health and Personal Social Services Statistics, 1982, Tables 3.23 and 3.24)

GENERAL DENTAL PRACTITIONERS

In 1981 there were in England:

- 12,835 general dental practitioners (GDP)
- 24,359 general medical practitioners
- 87 per cent of GDPs were male (but in those under 30 years of age 30 per cent were female)
- Persons per GDP in 1981: 3603 (in 1974 it was 1 GDP per 4192 persons)
- There were marked regional difference in distribution of GDPs
  - *1981* North West Thames (London) 1 per 2379
           Northern England   1 per 5002
  - *1974* North West Thames   1 per 2567
           Trent region   1 per 5916

(Source: *Health and Personal Social Services Statistics*, 1982, Tables 3.28 and 3.29)

LOCAL AUTHORITY SOCIAL SERVICES

Table 11   Local authority staff in social services

	Numbers	(WTE)
Social services		
Social workers	28,263	(26,641)
Administrators	22,281	(19,381)
Home helps	92,898	(48,809)
Others	135,748	(104,698)
Total	279,190	(199,529)
Residential homes		
For elderly	71,185	(52,535)
For children in care	26,912	(22,069)
For mental illness and handicap	9,189	(6,827)
Total	107,286	(81,431)
All	386,476	(280,960)

Source: *Health and Personal Social Services Statistics*, 1982, Table 3.32

In 1981 there were 386,476 staff employed by local authorities (=280,960 WTE). The distribution of these workers is shown in Table 11.

___

COMMENT

- The NHS is one of the largest *employers* with over 1 million staff. Of these only 3 per cent are GPs, 4 per cent hospital doctors (1.5 per cent are consultants) and 43 per cent are nurses and midwives. One half are non-medical or non-nursing.
- *Staff in NHS*, in relation to population, increased by a factor of 1.91 (1949–1981). Numbers of hospital doctors increased by 3.1 and GPs by 1.5. Nurses and midwives by 2.5. Administrators went up by 4.0 and paramedics and technicians by 4.5.
- Among *hospital doctors*, there are 8 male consultants to 1 female and 3 male junior hospital doctors to 1 female.
- *Foreign medical graduates* (overseas doctors) proportions in hospital grades:
  - consultants   17 per cent
  - senior registrars   25 per cent
  - registrars   50 per cent
  - senior house officers   46 per cent
  - pre-registration   12 per cent
- The *top specialties* in numbers of consultants are in order (in England):
  - all surgical
  - all medical
  - anaesthetics
  - psychiatrists
  - pathologists
  - radiologists
- There were 29,650 *general practitioners* in the NHS in 1982, including principals, assistants and trainees.
- In 1980 in the NHS there was 1 GP to 2017 persons, by 1990 it is likely to be 1 GP to 1834 persons.
- Four male GPs to 1 female.

- Twenty per cent of GPs are overseas doctors.
- *General dental practitioners*: half the number of general (medical) practitioners. Unevenly distributed.
- *Local authorities* employ 400,000 sociomedical staff.
- The *growth of NHS personnel* has shown a steady increase, almost 2-fold since the birth of the NHS. There are no manpower policies based on scientific operational data that include measurement and evaluation of quantity and quality of the work to be done.

CHAPTER 9

EDUCATION, TRAINING AND CAREERS

Table 1   Approximate annual entry to basic medical science courses in the United Kingdom. Medical schools, 1983

	Annual entry		Annual entry
Birmingham*	160	Manchester*	200
Bristol*	130	Newcastle*	130
Cambridge	210	Nottingham	130
Leeds*	160	Oxford	100
Leicester	100	Sheffield	150
Liverpool	150	Southampton	120
London:			
Charing Cross and			
Westminster	155	Belfast*	150
King's	105		
The London and			
St Bartholomew's†	210	Aberdeen*	130
Royal Free	100	Dundee*	110
St George's	140	Edinburgh	180
St Mary's	100	Glasgow	200
United Schools of Guy's and		St Andrews	80
St Thomas's	195		
University College and			
Middlesex†	195	Welsh National*	150

Source: Richards, P. (1983). *Br. Med. J.*, **287**, 409

*School offering a premedical (1st MB) course.

†Although The London and St Bartholomew's medical schools and University College and Middlesex medical schools are grouped together for the purposes of student entry quotas, they handle their admissions separately.

Between 1968 and 1978 the *number of medical students* increased by 36% from 2900 to 4600. The number of women increased by over 61% from 700 to 1800. In 1981, 43% of first-year

medical students and 41% of all applicants were women and the proportion is increasing.

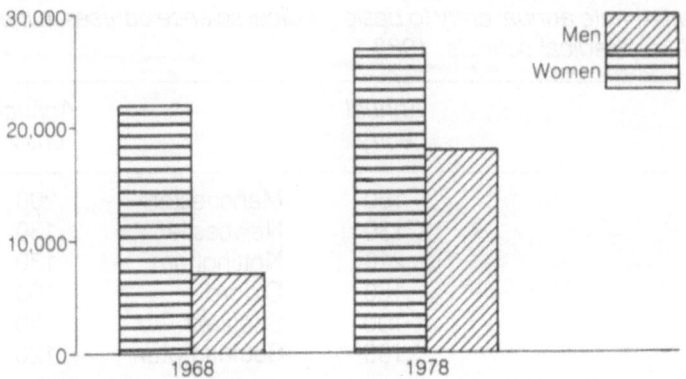

Figure 1   Number of medical students in training in years 1968 and 1978. Figures represent absolute numbers. Figures in parentheses express that number as a percentage of the total population of 18 year olds. (McManus, I. L. (1982). Br. Med. J., 284, 1654.)

Most medical schools admit between 120 and 150 students each year. In 1979–1980 the proportion of women admitted to medical schools varied between a low of 28% at the University of Wales to a high of 50% at the University of Bristol. However the proportion of women accepted is not fixed, and women do not necessarily have a better or worse chance of acceptance at any particular school.

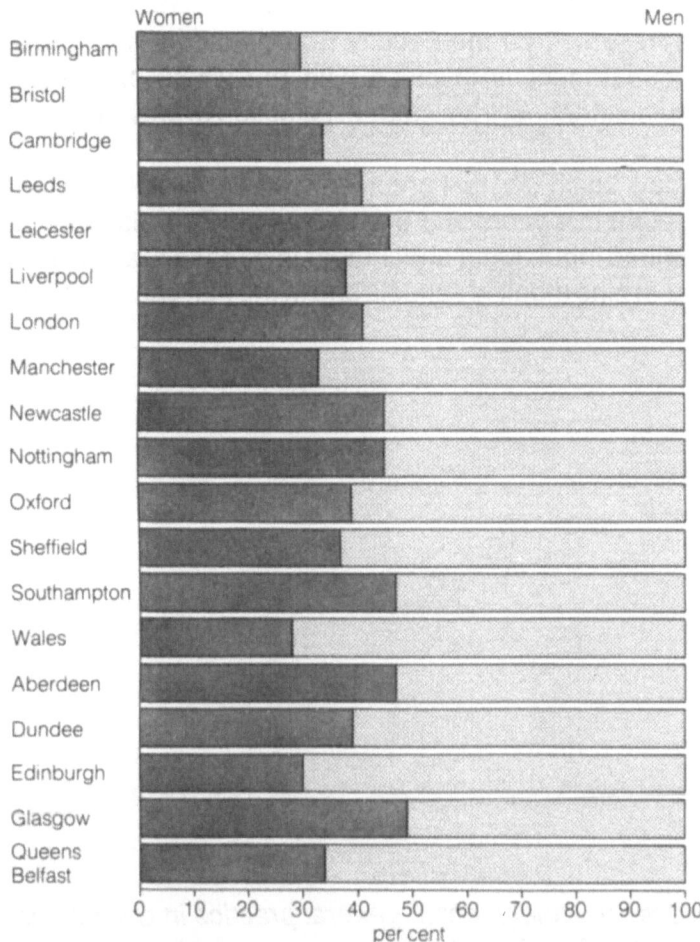

Figure 2 Women and men at different medical colleges, 1979–1980. Women as a percentage of the total number of students admitted to the medical curriculum. (GMC Education Committee)

MEDICAL SCHOOLS AND GENERAL PRACTICE

If Guy's and St Thomas's are considered separately there is organized general practice teaching in 27 out of 30 medical schools in the United Kingdom. Twelve have independent departments of general practice, ten headed by a professor. In 18 schools general practice is represented on the Faculty Board, and in 10 of these schools the department is involved with the whole process of running the medical school from student selection to providing final examiners.

Seven schools teach general practice in all 5 years of the standard course, eight in 4 years and five in 3 years. The rest provide much more limited input. Main attachment in general practice is in the fourth year in nine medical schools and in the fifth year in seven.

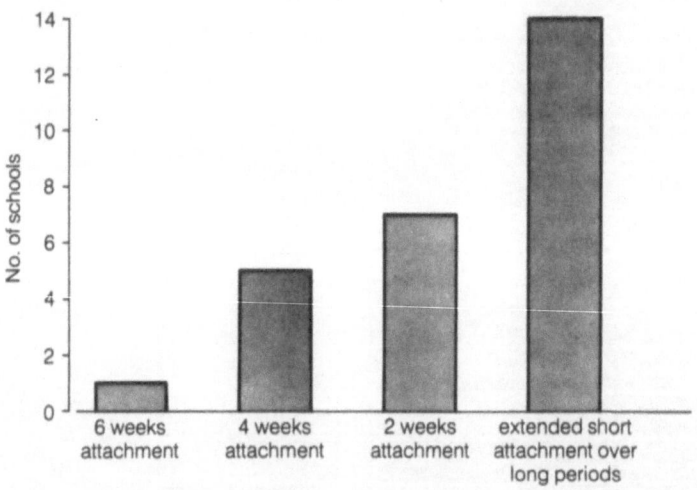

Figure 3   Weeks of attachment in general practice in UK medical schools (Metcalfe, D. (1980). Undergraduate teaching in general practice. In Fry, J. (ed.), Primary Care *(Heinemann, 1980).)*

COST OF MEDICAL TRAINING

The average net recurrent cost to universities of training a doctor in medicine between university entrance and MB graduation is an estimated £35,000 at 1980–1981 out-turn prices. Mandatory maintenance awards would be an additional £6000 per student.

NUMBERS OF SENIOR HOUSE OFFICER (SHO) POSTS

SHO posts are necessary for the general professional training of future consultants and general practitioners. The numbers of posts in Figure 4 demonstrate the surpluses and deficiencies in various specialties.

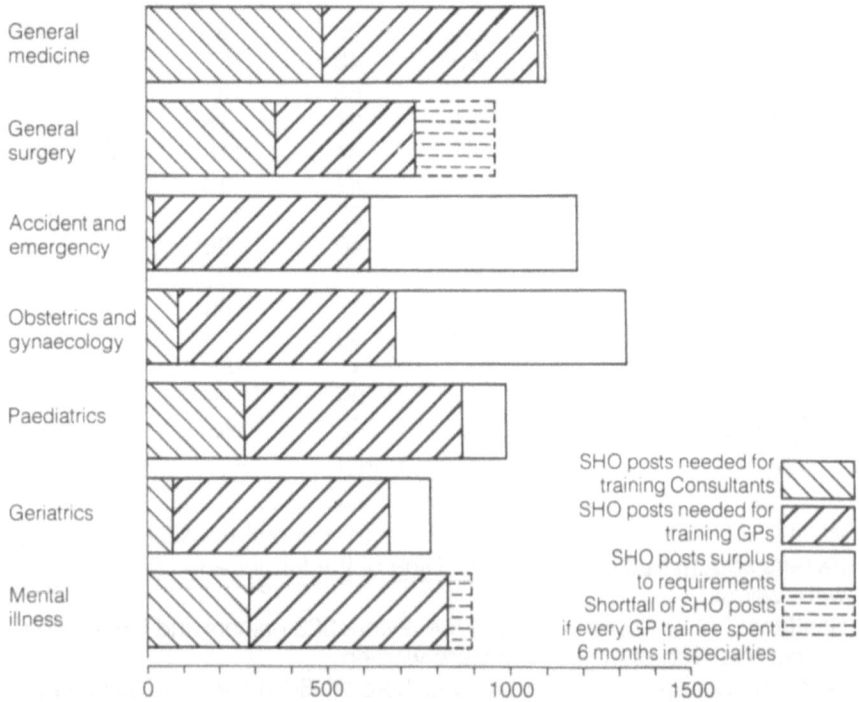

Figure 4   SHO posts in England and Wales, 1981 (Joint Committee on Postgraduate Training for General Practice)

VOCATIONAL TRAINING FOR GENERAL PRACTICE

Since 1982 there has been a mandatory 3-year training period for general practice. About one practice in four is recognized as a training practice. About 10% of all general practice principals are trainers. There was a 4-fold increase in trainers and a 7-fold increase in trainees between 1971 and 1981.

Table 2   Numbers of trainees and trainers in England, Wales, Scotland and Northern Ireland, 1981

England

Region	Trainees			Trainers (total)
	Men	Women	Total	
Northern	56	29	85	91
Yorkshire	59	46	105	138
Trent	79	56	135	189
East Anglia	51	27	78	114
North West Thames	74	44	118	153
North East Thames	71	47	118	155
South East Thames	54	33	113	162
South West Thames	54	40	94	116
Wessex	79	42	121	168
Oxford	47	19	66	94
South Western	86	39	125	173
West Midlands	106	47	153	133
Mersey	60	29	89	113
North Western	110	52	162	191
Total	1012	550	1562	2040

Wales   At 1 October 1981 there were 195 general medical practitioner trainers and 141 trainees in Wales. Nine of the former and 36 of the latter were women.

Scotland   At 30 September 1981 there were 306 trainers and 288 trainees in Scotland. Ten of the trainers were women.

Northern Ireland   In Northern Ireland there are 88 trainers and 53 trainees. Five of the trainees were women.

Source: *Br. Med. J.* (1982), **284**, 1420

Overall about one-third of general practitioner trainees are women. Trainers outnumber trainees because not all trainers have a trainee in post at any one time, and most regions observe a policy of appointing all suitable applicants.

POSTGRADUATE EXAMINATION PASS RATES

There are many postgraduate examinations in Britain. Their pass rates differ and are shown in Table 3.

Table 3   Pass rate of candidates in British postgraduate medical examinations 1978–1979

Specialty (all examinations)	Pass rate in first examination (percentage)	Pass rate in final examination (percentage)
Surgery		
British	43	45
Overseas	12	24
Medicine		
British	41	40
Overseas	25	21
General Practice		
British	—	66
Overseas	—	12
Obstetrics and gynaecology		
British	50	66
Overseas	30	33
Pathology		
British	66	59
Overseas	38	40
Psychiatry		
British	75	68
Overseas	32	38
Radiology		
British	77	38
Overseas	35	24
All subjects		
British	58	55
Overseas	28	27
PLAB		
Overseas	35	—

Source: *General Medical Council Annual Report*, 1982

CAREERS

There are approximately 45,000 senior posts available in the United Kingdom. There are approximately 25,000 general practitioners, 13,000 consultants and 7000 others (including specialists in community medicine). Approximately 55% of students will become general practitioners, and 28% consultants.

COMMENT

- The numbers of *medical students* increased by over one-third from 1968 to 1978, but the relationship to national manpower needs is uncertain.
- *General practice undergraduate teaching* is carried out in almost all medical schools. The arrangements are variable.
- The *cost* of training a medical student till graduation in 1980/1981 was £41,000.
- *Vocational training for GPs* is now mandatory, and involves one-quarter of all general practices. One in 10 of GPs is an approved trainer.
- *Pass rates for postgraduate final examinations* show average of 55 per cent for UK graduates and 27 per cent for overseas doctors. Surgery, medicine and radiology have lower pass rates than general practice, OBG, pathology and psychiatry.

CHAPTER 10

UTILIZATION OF RESOURCES AND CONTENT OF WORK

UTILIZATION

There are three sectors of utilization of health care:

● self-care;
● primary professional care (general practice in NHS);
● hospital care.

Figure 1 is a representation of the proportions of symptoms dealt with at each of these.

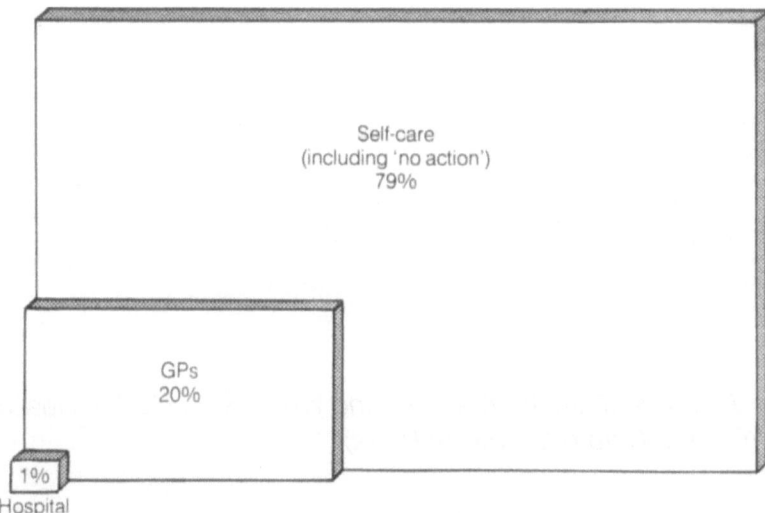

Figure 1 Symptoms: proportions cared at self-care, general practice and hospital levels (percentages of symptoms) (Fry, J. (1978). A New Approach to Medicine (Lancaster: MTP))

SELF-TREATMENT

State of health

At any time the state of health in the community is as shown in Figure 2:

● healthy+   13 per cent
● not-ill (well)   52 per cent
● ill   18 per cent
● chronic sickness   12 per cent
● disabled   5 per cent

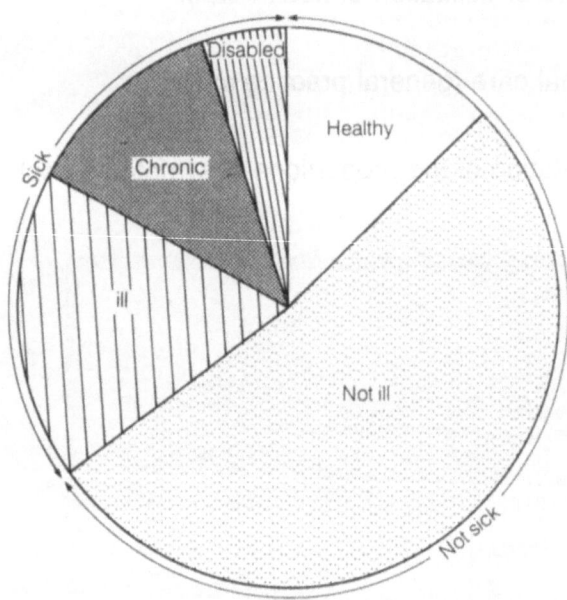

Figure 2 State of health (Kohn, R. and White, K. L. (1976). Health Care. *(Oxford: Oxford University Press))*

What do they do when sick?

When persons develop symptoms their actions are likely to be as shown in Figure 3:

130   UTILIZATION OF RESOURCES

- no action   16 per cent
- self-medication   63 per cent
- visit GP   20 per cent
- go to hospital   1 per cent

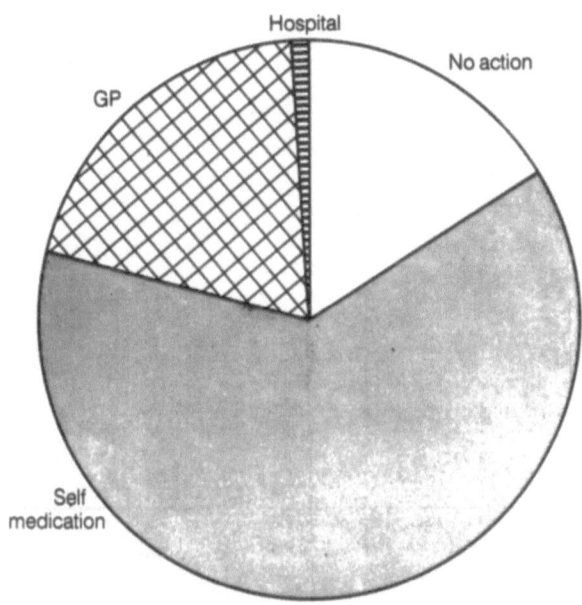

Figure 3 Sickness – action taken (Fry, J. (1978). A New Approach to Medicine. *(Lancaster: MTP))*

Medication

At any time 60 per cent of the population is likely to be taking some medicine on any day (Figure 4). Of this:

- 27 per cent will be prescribed medicines;
- 33 per cent will be non-prescribed medicines (self-medication);

(Kohn, R. and White, K. L. *op cit.*, 1976)

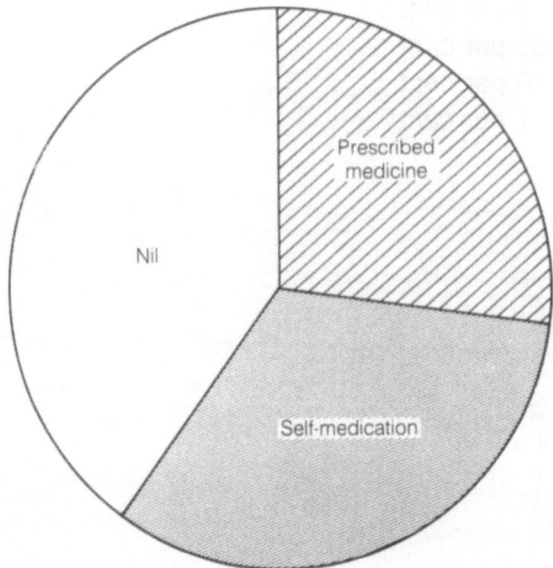

Figure 4   Medication in population

GENERAL PRACTICE

Contacts with general practitioner (Figure 5)

- when persons have symptoms one-fifth will visit their general practitioner.
- *in any year*
  approximately two-thirds of all persons in UK will consult their GP, one or more times.
- *in a period of 5 years*
  approximately 90 per cent will have consulted their GP, the likely contact-rate between GP and his patients is very high.

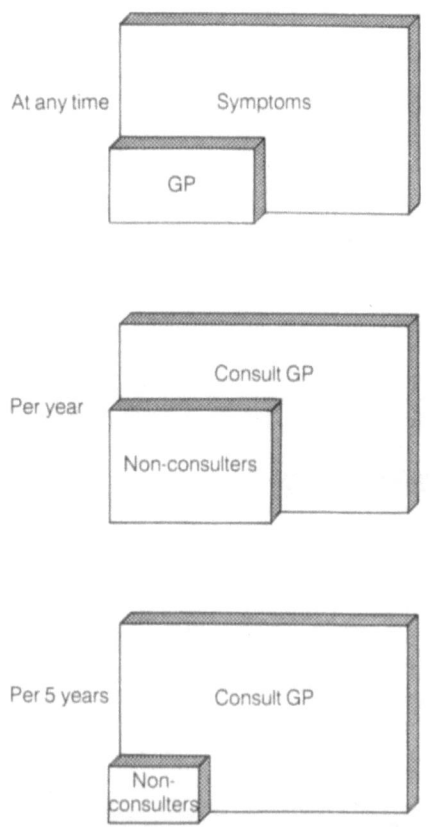

Figure 5   Contacts with a general practitioner

Annual consultation rates

A measure of utilization is the annual consultation rate per person. The mean rate in the NHS is *between 3.5 and 4.0 consultations per year* (National Morbidity Surveys and General Household Surveys.)

Sex: The rate is higher in females (4.4) than males (3.3) (Figure 6).
Age: The highest consultation rates are in infants and in old age (Figure 7).

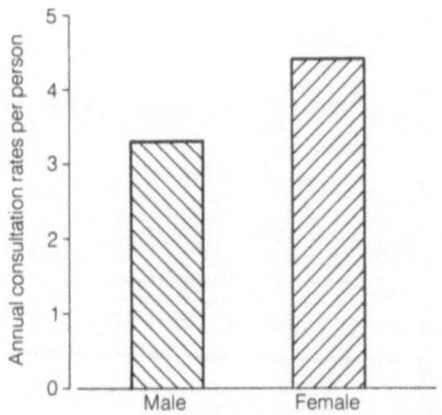

Figure 6   Annual consultation rates by sex

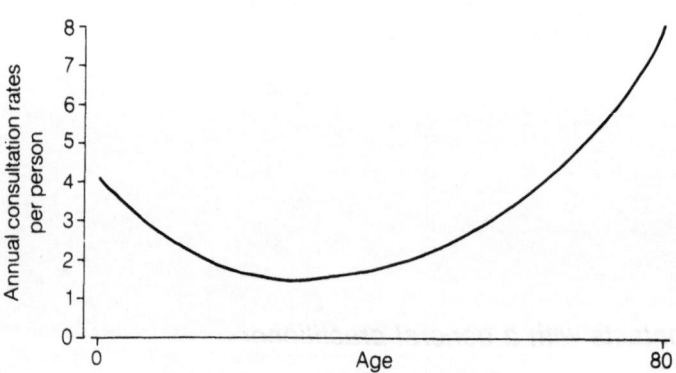

Figure 7   Annual consultation rates by age

GP work profile

In a practice with 2500 persons NHS registered the likely *work profile* (Figure 8) is:

- surgery consultations   30–40 per day
- home visits   3–4 per day
- night visits   1 every 2 weeks

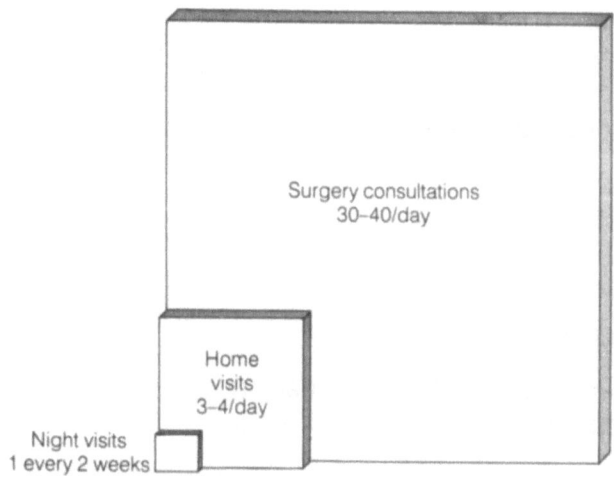

Figure 8   GP work profile

Another way of expressing division of GP work and utilization is by
the various activities (Figure 9):

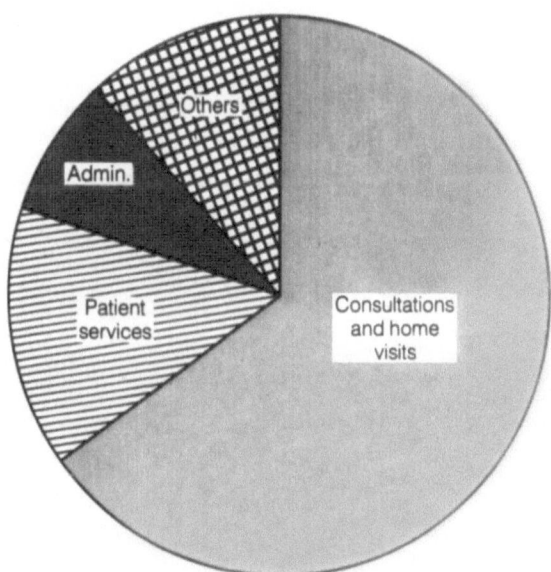

*Figure 9   General practice – allocation of work/utilization (RCGP
(1983).* Present State and Future Needs. *(Lancaster: MTP))*

- consultations and home visits — 65 per cent
- patient services (letters, phone, prescriptions) — 15 per cent
- practice administration — 8 per cent
- other professional activities — 12 per cent

General practice referrals to hospital

In a practice of 2500 persons the annual numbers of persons referred to, or utilizing, hospital services will be:

In-patients
- 275 discharges/deaths:
    - surgical   140
    - medical   80
    - obstetric   30
    - others   25

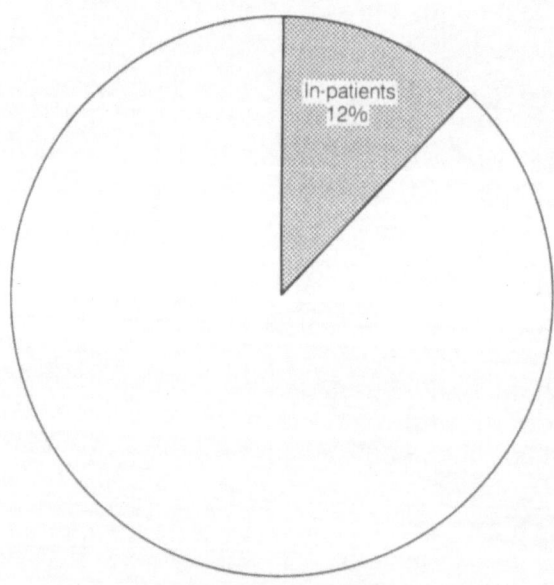

Figure 10   GP: annual hospital admissions (per 100 population)

Outpatients
- 415 new referrals to outpatient departments

surgical	250
medical	110
obstetric	30
others	25

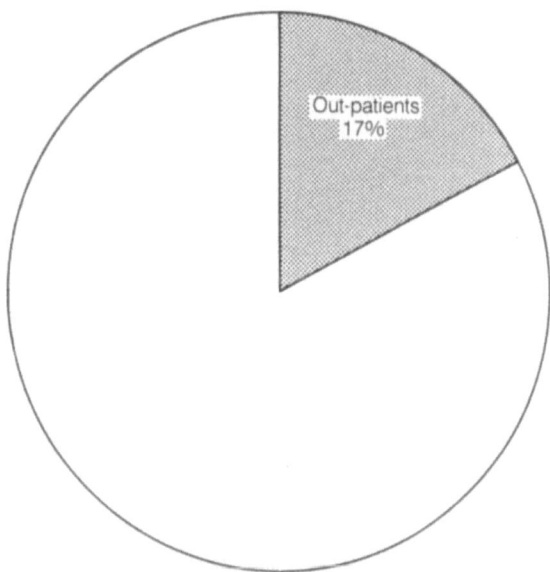

Figure 11   GP: annual new referrals to outpatient departments (per 100 population)

Thus, it is likely that about 20 per cent of all persons will be referred to outpatient departments and/or admitted – some will use both services. This represents only 5 per cent of GP consultations. 1 in 5 will be treated in hospital (plus others in accident–emergency departments), but in only 1 general practice consultation in 20 will referral be made.

Domiciliary consultations:

- In any year a GP will arrange *18 'domiciliary consultations'* by a consultant.

- The mean annual numbers of *domiciliary consultations per consultant will be 36.*
- The top four specialties of domiciliary consultations per consultant in the various specialties (Figure 12) are:
  - geriatrics   217
  - mental illness   91
  - medicine   78
  - surgery   54

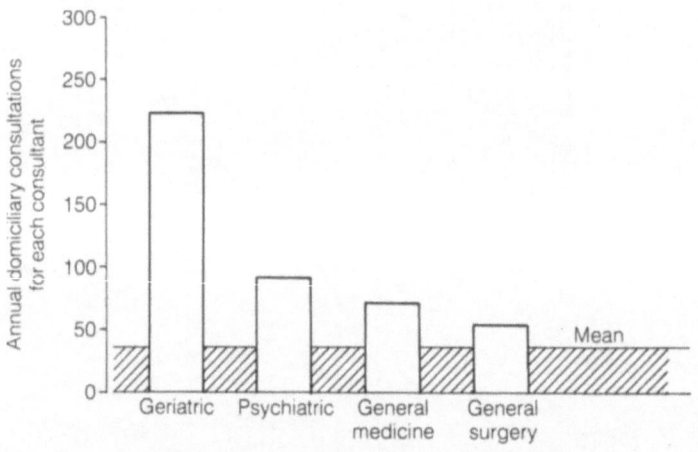

Figure 12 Annual domiciliary consultations per consultant in various specialties: mean numbers (Personal data, DHSS)

DIAGNOSTIC SERVICES

Use of Pathology and Radiology

The use of pathology and radiology resources increases annually (Figure 13). The rises between 1958 and 1977 have been 3–4-fold. By 1983 it is likely to have been 6-fold.

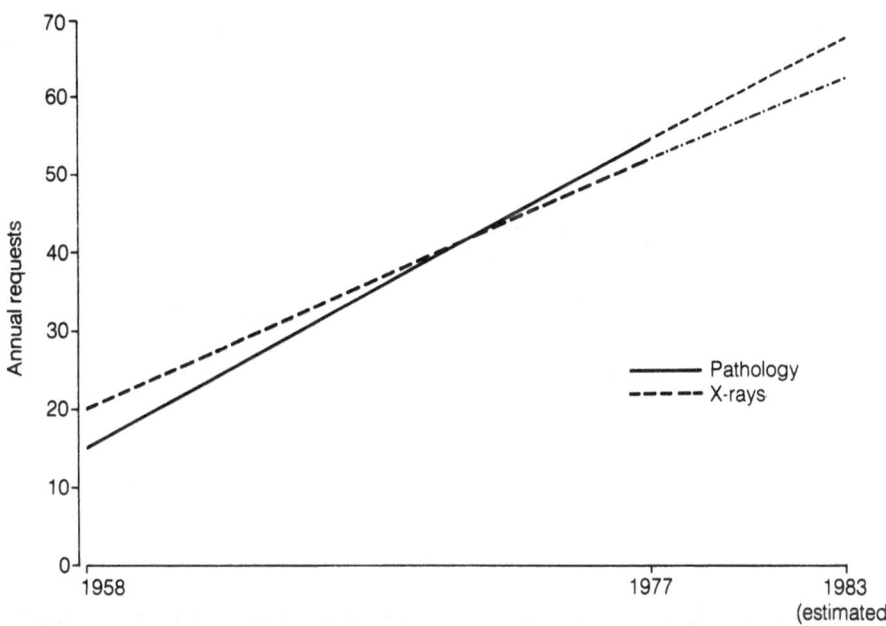

Figure 13   Numbers of pathology and radiology requests in NHS (1958–1977) (From Health and Personal Social Services Statistics, *1978)*

HOSPITAL SERVICES

Utilization rates

Figure 14 and Table 1 show the rates per 1000 of hospital resources (beds allocated) and those treated as inpatients, outpatients and as accidents–emergencies. Beds allocated have fallen, and utilization of services has increased.

Table 1   NHS hospitals: utilization rates (per 1000 population)

	1949	*1959*	*1969*	*1979*
Allocated hospital beds	10.3	10.6	9.5	8.0
Inpatients	67	88	109	117
Outpatients (new referrals)	140	159	166	167
Accident–emergency (new cases)	89	121	166	198

Source: *Health and Personal Social Services Statistics,* 1982, Tables 4.3 and 4.6

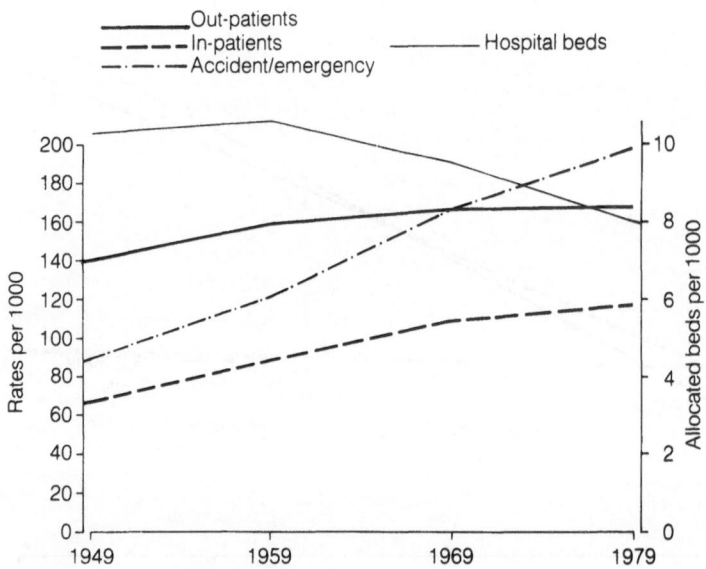

Figure 14 NHS hospitals: utilization rates (per 1000 population)
(Health and Personal Social Services Statistics, *1982, Tables 4.3 and 4.6)*

In a year (1979) the proportions of the population using medical resources were as shown in Figure 15:

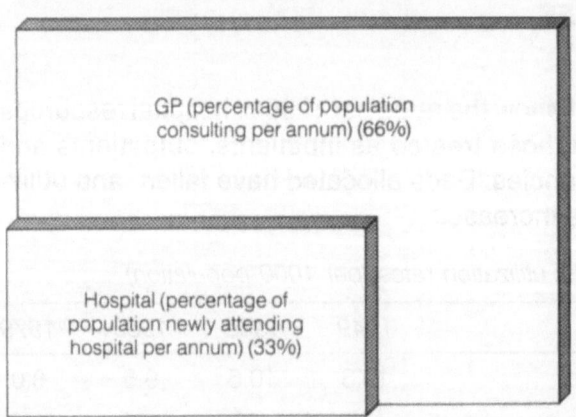

GP (percentage of population consulting per annum) (66%)

Hospital (percentage of population newly attending hospital per annum) (33%)

Figure 15   Annual utilization of medical services (per 100 persons)

- inpatients   12 per cent
- (new) outpatients   17 per cent

- (new) accident–emergency   20 per cent
- approximate all persons attending hospitals   33 per cent
- consulting GP   66 per cent

Note that there are four outpatient department attendances for each new outpatient, so that the proportion of all persons attending hospitals is higher than the approximate 33 per cent in Figure 15 because some 'old' outpatients attend over many years.

Length of hospital stay

The mean lengths of stay in hospital have been falling (Figure 16 and Table 2).

Table 2   *Hospitals: mean length of stay* (1970–1980)*

	1970	1975	1980
Mean number of days	11.3	10.2	8.3
Base 1970 = 100	100	88	70

*Non-psychiatric specialties and excluding geriatrics and units for the younger disabled
Source: *Personal Social Services Statistics*, 1982, Table 4.6

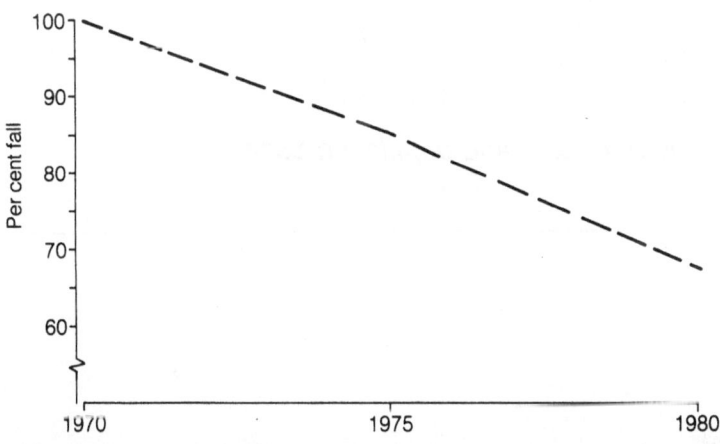

Figure 16   *Hospitals: mean lengths of stay (1970–1980) (non-psychiatric specialties and excluding geriatrics and units for younger disabled)* (Health and Personal Social Services Statistics, 1982, Table 4.6)

CLINICAL CONTENT

The clinical content at the three levels of care is different in emphasis. It is important to appreciate these differences as they influence management and education. The differences are partly because of the selection of the clinical material and the patterns of referrals but they also relate to the different population bases (Figure 17). Thus:

- *self-care* will be in the context of a family unit of 1–10 persons;
- *general practice:* with approximately 2500 per GP;
- a *district general hospital* providing care for about 250,000 persons.

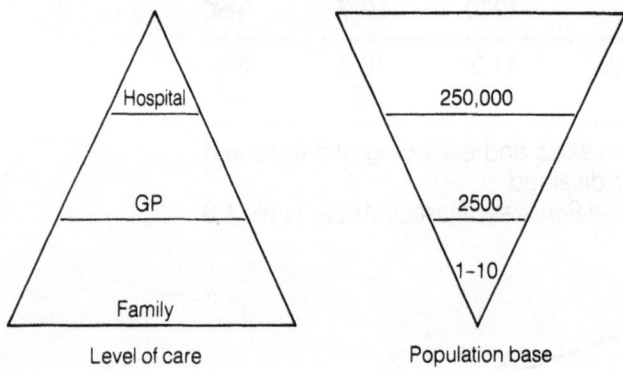

Figure 17   Levels of care and population bases

SELF-CARE

Precise medical diagnoses are not possible at the level of self-care. It is on *symptoms* that their interpretation and treatment is based. The most prevalent symptoms in the community are shown in Figure 18 and Table 3.

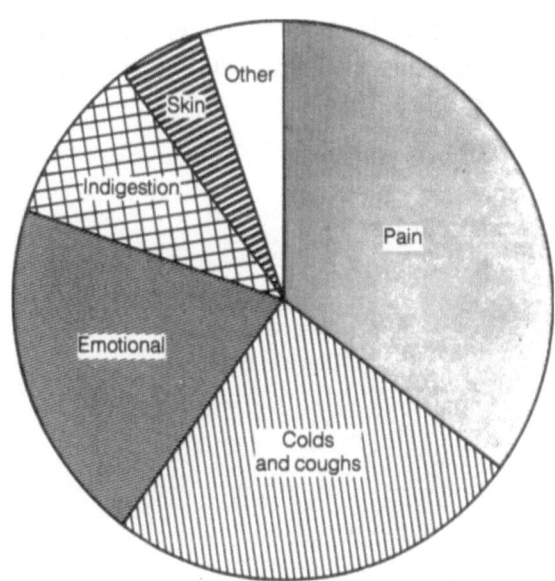

Figure 18 Self-care: percentages of common symptoms (Fry, J. (1978). A New Approach to Medicine, op. cit.)

Table 3   Self-care: common symptoms

Symptoms	Percentage of symptoms requiring self-care
Pain (headache, backache, painful limbs)	35
Coughs and colds	25
Emotional (low state, anxiety, tension)	20
Flatulence, indigestion, dyspepsia	10
Skin rashes	5
Others	5

Source: Fry, J. *(1978)*. A New Approach to Medicine, *op. cit.*

GENERAL PRACTICE (see also Chapter 3)

In the NHS general practice is the first level of professional care. It provides care for conditions that can be managed in the community. It protects the hospital services from inappropriate patients, and patients from inappropriate hospitals.

The bulk of the clinical material is with relatively *minor* (non-serious and self-limiting) conditions and with *chronic* (persistent and non-curable) disorders (Figure 19):

- minor conditions   65 per cent
- chronic disorders   20 per cent
- acute major diseases   15 per cent

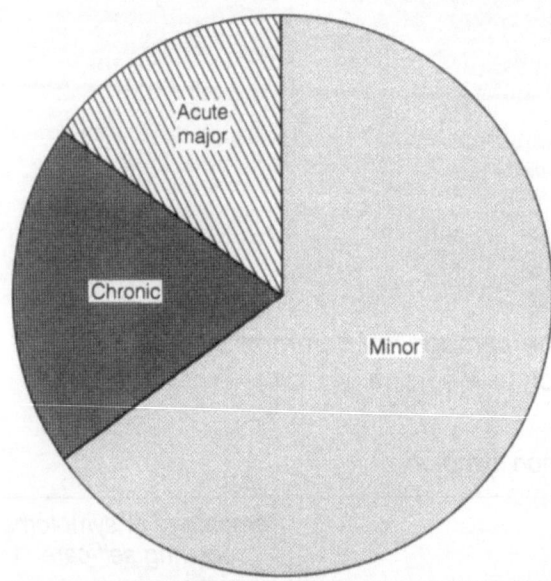

Figure 19 General practice: grades of disease (Fry, J. (1983). Common Diseases, *3rd edition, op. cit.)*

Table 4 Minor conditions: general classification

General classification	Annual persons consulting per 2500
Upper respiratory conditions	600
Skin disorders	350
Psycho-emotional	250
Minor accidents	250
Gastro-intestinal	200
Rheumatic	150
'Symptoms'	375

The approximate numbers of persons consulting their GP with a practice of 2500 patients in a year are shown in Tables 4–9 for minor, chronic and acute major (life-threatening) conditions. Social pathologies also are shown (data from Fry, J., *op. cit.*).

Table 5   Minor conditions: specific diagnoses

Specific diagnosis	Annual persons consulting per 2500
Acute throat infections	100
Eczema–dermatitis	100
Acute otitis media	75
Ear wax	50
Urinary tract infections	50
Acute backache	50
Vaginal discharge	30
Migraine	25
Hay fever	25
Vertigo (dizziness)	20
Hernia	10
Piles	10

Table 6   Chronic disorders

Specific diagnosis	Annual persons consulting per 2500
High blood pressure	250
Chronic arthritis	200
Chronic psycho-emotional	100
Ischaemic heart disease	50
Cardiac failure	40
Cancers (all stages)	30
Diabetes	30
Asthma	30
Peptic ulcers	25
Strokes (all stages)	20
Thyroid disorders	10
Epilepsy	10
Multiple sclerosis	3
Parkinsonism	3
End renal failure	(less than) 1

Table 7   Acute major diseases

Diagnosis	Annual persons consulting per 2500

Acute chest infections
   (acute bronchitis: 100)
   (pneumonia: 20)
	120

Severe depression
   (parasuicide: 5)
   (suicide: 1 every 4 years)
	10

Acute myocardial infarction (sudden death: 5)	10
Acute strokes	6
New cancers	6
Acute abdominal emergencies (appendicitis: 4)	6

Table 8   Some new cancers

Site	Annual persons consulting per 2500
All new cancers	6
Lung – bronchus	2
Breast	1
Large bowel	2 every 3 years
Stomach	1 every 2 years
Prostate	1 every 3 years
Bladder	1 every 3 years
Cervix	1 every 4 years
Ovary	1 every 6 years
Oesophagus	1 every 7 years
Brain	1 every 10 years
Lymphadenoma	1 every 10 years
Leukaemia	1 every 10 years

Table 9   Social pathologies

Condition	Likely prevalence per 2500
Poverty	
'Poor' receiving supplementary benefits	120
Unemployed	100 +
Marriage, etc.	
Marriage per year	12
Divorce per year	3
One-parent families	40
Crime	
Burglaries per year	25
Adults in prison	4
Juvenile delinquents	10
Children in care	3
Drunken driving	5
Sexual assault	1

HOSPITAL (see also Chapter 3)

It is more difficult to provide such detailed comprehensive data from the hospital level, but piecemeal there follow some facts from a variety of sources.

Inpatients (discharges and deaths)

A modern urban district general hospital provides care for approximately 250,000 persons. With an annual inpatient rate of 12 per cent the numbers being admitted to that hospital will be 30,000.

The hospital inpatient enquiry for 1982 (HIPE 1982) provides data from which approximate annual numbers of patients in some clinical categories might be expected to be admitted (Table 10).

Table 10   District general hospital annual admissions (250,000 population base)

Diagnostic group		Annual hospital admissions per 250,000 (deaths and discharges)	Percentage
All admissions		30,000	100
Injuries and poisoning		2800	10
(fractures	900)		
(parasuicide	500)		
'Symptoms'		2650	9
(abdominal pain	550)		
Cardiovascular		2600	9
(myocardial infarction	620)		
(strokes	575)		
(hypertension	100)		
(other heart conditions	520)		
(varicose veins	150)		
(piles	400)		
Gastro-intestinal		2500	8
(hernia	500)		
(appendicitis	400)		
(gall bladder	300)		
(peptic ulcer	200)		
Neoplasms		1500	5
(lung-bronchus	250)		
(breast	200)		
(bladder	200)		
(lymphatic	200)		
(benign	400)		
Respiratory		1950	7
(chronic airways disease	500)		
(pneumonia	350)		
(tonsillectomy	400)		
Others		16,000	51

Source: Hospital Inpatient Enquiry (HIPE), 1982 (HMSO)

Hospital admissions per consultant

Translating these large numbers to expectations that a consultant may expect in a year gives the results shown in Table 11 and Figure 20.

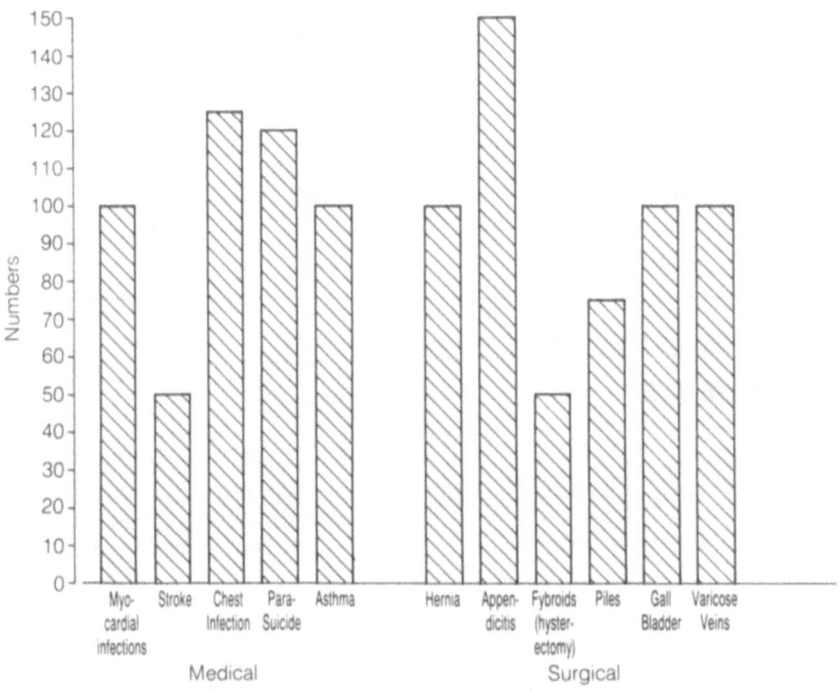

Figure 20 Annual hospital admissions per consultant (common diagnoses) (HIPE, 1982)

Table 11 Annual hospital admissions per consultant (common diagnoses)

Diagnosis	Annual admissions per consultant
Medical	
Acute chest infections	100
Acute asthma	50
Acute myocardial infarctions	125
Acute strokes	120
Parasuicide	100
Surgical	
Appendicitis	100
Hernia	150
Varicose veins	50
Gall bladder	75
Piles	100
Fibroids (hysterectomy)	100
Cancer of lung–bronchus	50
Peptic ulcers	60

Source: *HIPE*, 1982

OUTPATIENTS

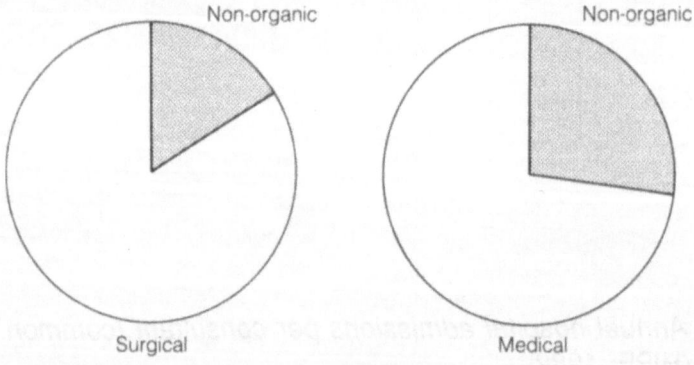

Figure 21 Hospital outpatients: non-organic diagnoses in percentages (Forsyth, G. and Logan, R. (1968). Gateway or Dividing Line. (Oxford University Press for Nuffield Provincial Hospitals Trust))

Data for content of outpatient attendances is scanty. Forsyth and Logan (1968) provide an insight. The content by percentages of diagnoses is shown in Table 12 and Figure 21.

Table 12   Hospital outpatients: diagnoses (percentages)

Diagnostic group	Percentage of diagnoses
General surgical	
Nil abnormal found, no diagnosis or mental-psychiatric	16
Malignant neoplasms	6
Benign neoplasms	7
Varicose veins	7
Piles	4
Hernia	13
Gastro-intestinal	12
Skin	8
General medical	
Nil abnormal found, no diagnosis, or mental-psychiatric	27
Neoplasms	3
Endocrine	12
CNS	7
CVS	17
Respiratory	5
Gastro-intestinal	10
Rheumatic	5

Source: Forsyth, G. and Logan, R., *op. cit.*

COMMENT

- Of all persons who are *unwell with symptoms*:
  - 79 per cent will apply self-care, which includes 'no action';
  - 20 per cent will visit their GP;
  - 1 per cent will be seen at hospital.

- *At any time:*
  - 13 per cent are 'healthy';
  - 60 per cent will be taking medicines, of which one-half are non-prescribed.
- *General practice:*
  - Two-thirds of the population will consult their GP in any year.
  - Nine-tenths will consult their GP in 5 years.
- A *typical day in general practice* will include:
  - 30–40 surgery consultations
  - 3–4 home visits
  - 1 night visit every 2 weeks
- *Hospital referrals* by a GP:
  - 1 in 20 of consultations
  - 1 in 5 of all persons seen
- *Domiciliary consultations:*
  - 18 per year per GP
  - 36 per year per consultant
- The top specialties claiming for domiciliary consultations are (per year):
  - geriatrics   217
  - psychiatry   91
  - general medicine   78
  - general surgery   54
- *Hospital utilization* – each year:
  - 12 per cent of the population is admitted to hospital;
  - 17 per cent of the population is newly referred by GPs to outpatient departments (each new OP will average four attendances);
  - 20 per cent of the population attend accident–emergency departments.
- It is likely that one-third of the population will receive some *hospital care* in a year.
- The average *stay in hospital* is 8 days; this is a reduction of 30 per cent since 1970.
- The *content of general practice* is predominantly minor and chronic disorders.
- The spectrum of *content* of *hospital practice* has a large segment of 'common diseases' related to the particular specialty.

What is 'common' in neurosurgery certainly is not common in general surgery.

- Data on *utilization* of *medical resources* are piecemeal and incomplete.
- If *optimal use* is to be made of available resources then much more attention must be paid not only to use of resources in general, but also to utilization profiles of separate hospitals, of specialist and general practice units and of individual consultants and practitioners.
- *Utilization rates* must be related also to the content and nature of the disorders being treated.

CHAPTER 11

PRESCRIBING

Taking of drugs by individuals, and prescribing of drugs by doctors, are normal and inevitable activities. They occur in all societies and in all countries. At any time and on any day probably 60 per cent of the population are taking medicinal drugs. Kohn and White, *op. cit.* (1976) found this rate in 12 developed countries (Figure 1). Of these one-half will be drugs prescribed by doctors and one-half self-medicated by purchasing medicines 'over the counter' (OTC).

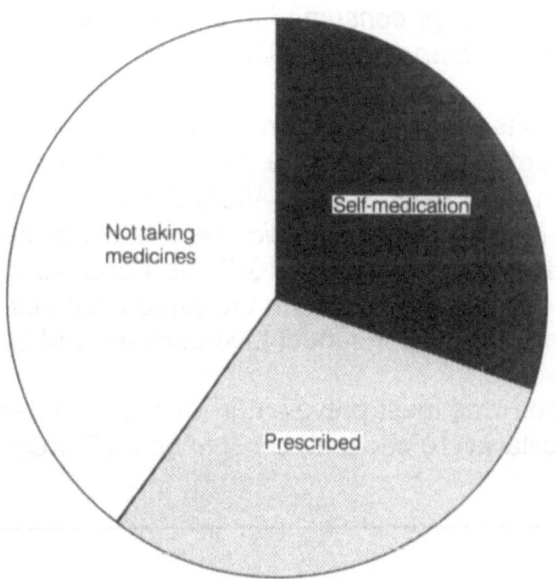

Figure 1 Medication in a developed country – percentage taking medicines at any time (after Kohn and White, 1976)

SELF-MEDICATION (OTC drugs)

The groups of OTC drugs most widely consumed are analgesics, vitamins and cough medicines (Figure 2).

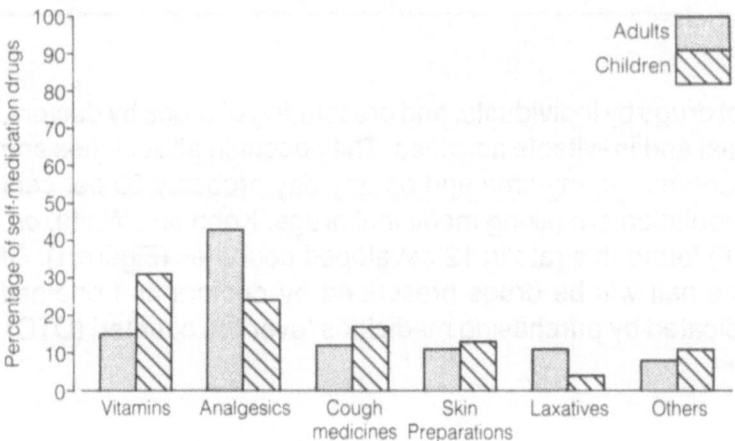

Figure 2   Self-medication drugs consumed in any day (percentage of population) (after Kohn and White, 1976)

There are national habits of self-medication. Thus *vitamins* were consumed by 59 per cent of children and 29 per cent of adults in Helsinki compared with 8 per cent (Buenos Aires) and 2 per cent (Yugoslavia) of adults respectively. *Analgesics* were taken by 69 per cent of Yugoslav adults and by 33 per cent of Finns. For children the rates were 61 per cent and 7 per cent in the same countries. *Laxatives* were consumed by 16 per cent of Liverpudlians and by 2 per cent of Yugoslavs.

Overall self-medication was most prevalent in Canada (40 per cent) and least in Yugoslavia (10 per cent) consuming OTC drugs at any time.

PRESCRIBED DRUGS IN NHS

Costs of drugs have been at around 10 per cent of total cost of the NHS ever since 1949. In 1983 the cost of the NHS will be over £15,000 million and that of drugs almost £1500 million (Figure 3).

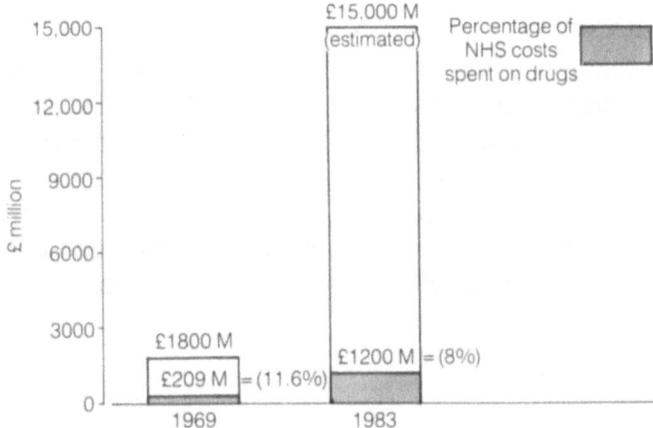

Figure 3   Cost of NHS 1969 and 1983, and percentages of costs of drugs

General practitioner prescriptions make up three-quarters of all drug costs in the NHS (Figure 4).

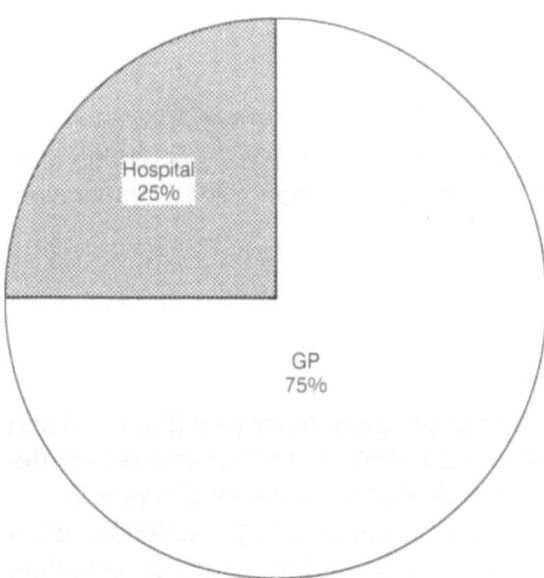

Figure 4   Proportions of costs of drugs in NHS – by hospital doctors and by GPs

Prescribing costs per GP

The annual prescribing costs per GP are about twice his NHS income. Thus in 1983 his prescribing costs will be around £50,000 and his income approximately £23,000. The prescribing costs per GP from 1949 to 1983 reveal that taking into account inflationary trends in real terms (1949 prices) the cost of GP prescriptions increased by 4.75 fold (Figure 5). The average cost for each GP prescription now in 1983 is £4.00. In 1949 it was 16 pence.

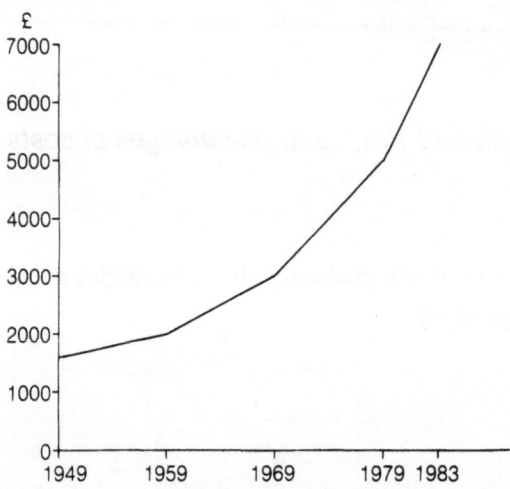

Figure 5 Annual expenditure per GP on NHS prescriptions in 1949 constant prices (Office of Health Economics Compendium (OHE), 1981)

Volume of prescriptions

The volume of GP prescriptions per person per year (Figure 6) and per GP shows an increase from 1969 to 1979 and a recent decrease, possibly because of the higher prescription charges. These rates imply that each GP will write out 14,000 prescriptions each year, or 40–45 each working day. Since the annual consultation rate per person is 3.5–4 per year it means that almost one-half of all prescriptions are for 'non-consultations', i.e. for repeat or other reasons.

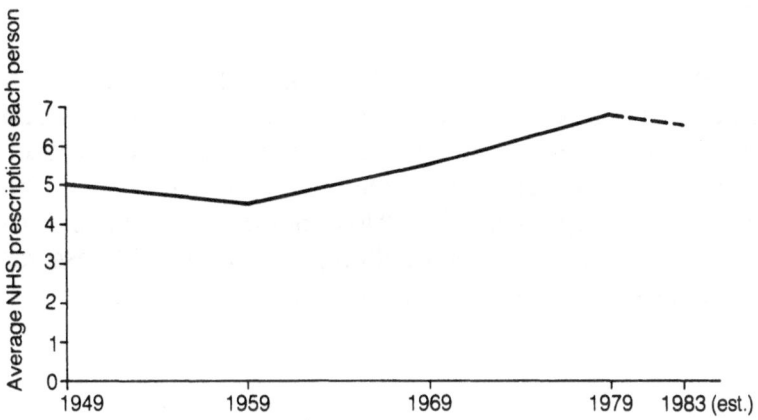

Figure 6   Annual number of prescriptions per person in NHS
(Health and Personal Social Services Statistics, *1982, Table 5.9, and*
other personal data from DHSS)

Lest it be thought that the annual number of prescriptions per
person is high in the NHS Figure 7 shows comparable rates in other
European countries.

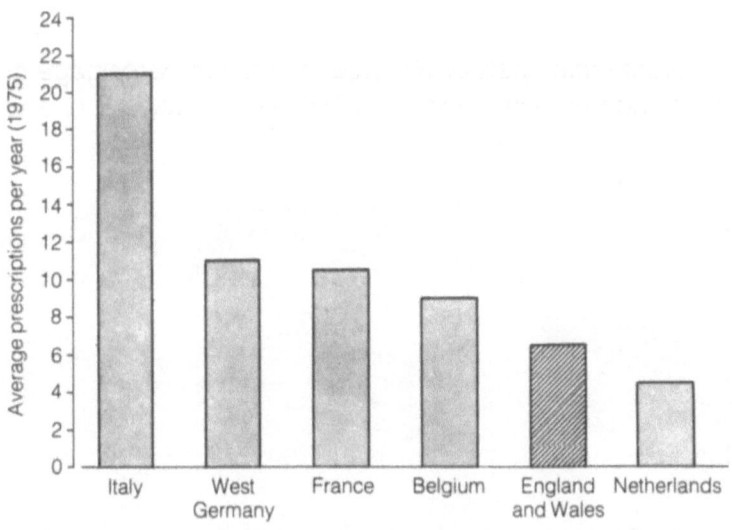

Figure 7   Annual number of prescriptions issued per person in
some European countries in 1975 (Office of Health Economics,
personal information)

What is prescribed?

The therapeutic groups of drugs prescribed by GPs and their relative costs in Figure 8 show that the most frequently prescribed drugs were for nervous system disorders, for cardiovascular drugs, antibiotics, and for respiratory conditions. In terms of costs the drugs that were expensive in relation to their frequency of use were the cardiovascular and rheumatic therapeutic groups. Those for the nervous system were relatively cheaper.

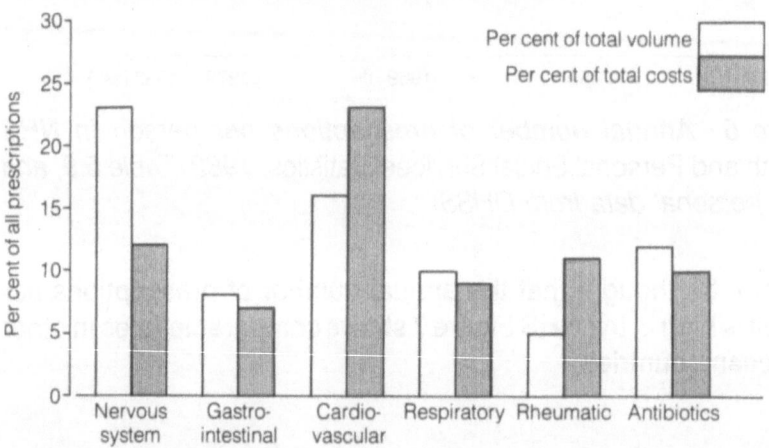

Figure 8 Volume and costs of GP prescriptions in percentage of totals (Health and Personal Social Statistics, *1982, Tables 5.11 and 5.12)*

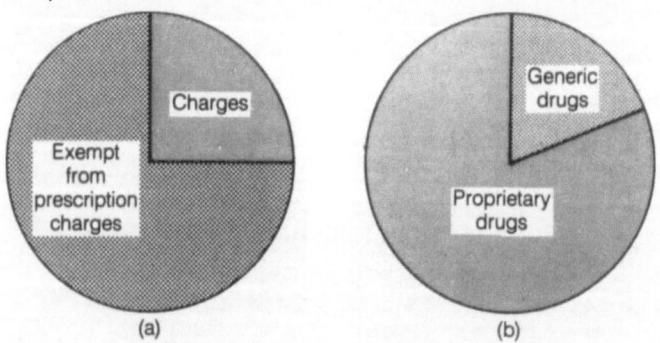

Figure 9 (a) Percentages who are exempt from prescription charges; (b) percentages of prescriptions for proprietary and generic drugs (Health and Personal Social Services Statistics, *1982, Tables 5.9 and 5.10)*

Note that of all prescriptions 75 per cent were exempt from a prescription charge and 81 per cent were for proprietary drugs (Figure 9a, b).

Dispensing doctors

Within the NHS 8 per cent of general practitioners (2247 in 1980) are dispensing doctors in rural areas. They dispense their own prescriptions and are allowed to make profits on the transactions.

There are marked differences and costs in the annual rates of prescriptions per dispensing GP compared with his non-dispensing colleagues (Figure 10).

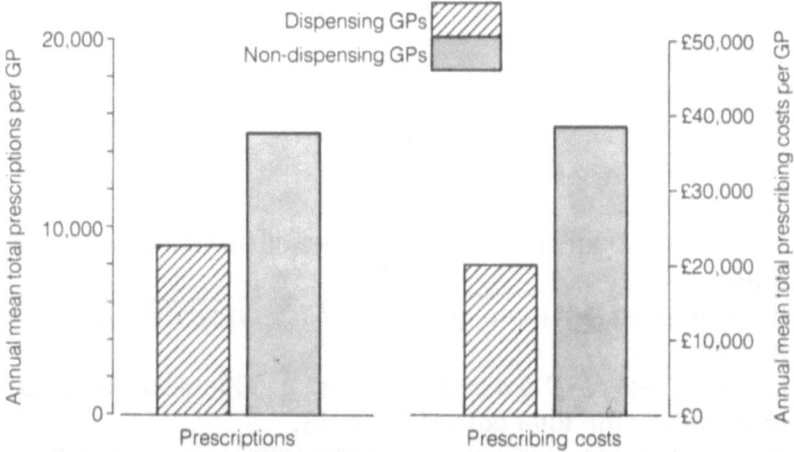

Figure 10   Dispensing and non-dispensing GPs – mean total prescriptions and total prescribing costs (1981) (OHE Compendium, Tables 4.11 and 4.16)

Chemists establishments

The numbers of chemist shops (establishments) is being reduced each year (Figure 11). The single-handed chemist is disappearing and is being replaced by supermarket type of establishment, just as the solo GP is being replaced by the group practice.

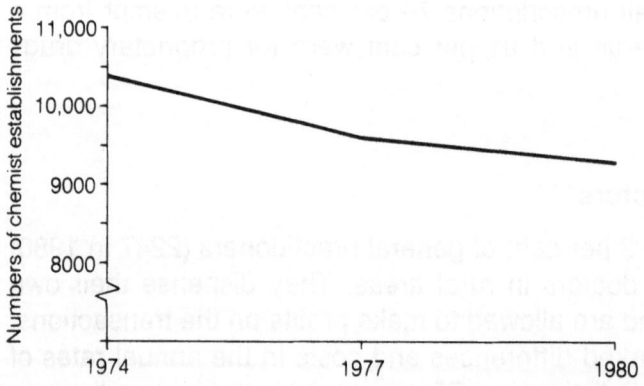

Figure 11 Number of chemists establishments in England, 1974–1980 (Health and Personal Social Services Statistics, *1982*, Chart 5.7)

COMMENT

- At any time about one-third of persons will be taking *prescribed drugs*.
- It is estimated that three-quarters of *NHS prescribing costs* are by GPs.
- In 1983 GPs' *NHS prescriptions cost* £1500 million or almost one-tenth of the total cost of the NHS.
- On average each *GP prescribed* £50,000 of drugs in 1983.
- At constant (1949) prices the *cost of GP prescribing* has increased by a factor of 4.75.
- The *annual rate of 6–7 NHS prescriptions* per person may appear high but is much less than rates of 21 in Italy and 11 in West Germany and France.
- The most widely *prescribed drugs* are analgesics and psychotropics, drugs for cardiovascular diseases, antibiotics and antirheumatics.
- There are large differences in *prescribing rates and costs* between NHS regions and between individual GPs. It is likely that savings to the NHS could be made in this field.

CHAPTER 12

PSYCHIATRY

At present (1983) some 160 per 100,000 or 1.6 per cent of the UK population are in NHS psychiatric hospitals. In a year only 40 per 100,000 or 1 in 4 are discharged, indicating that many inmates are long-stay residents.

Proportions of resources

In 1980 in England more than one-half of all hospital beds were psychiatric beds (Figure 1 and Table 1). The discharge rate was low, and new referrals to outpatient departments were low also.

Table 1   Hospital psychiatric resources per 100,000 (England, 1980) and as percentages of total service

Inpatients	Occupied beds	Discharges and deaths
All specialties	7.7	122
Non-psychiatric	3.7	118
Psychiatric	4.0	4
	(52%)	(3%)

Outpatients	New referrals to OPD
All specialties	171
Non-psychiatric	161
Psychiatric	10 (6%)

Source: *Health and Personal Social Services Statistics*, 1982, Table 4.4

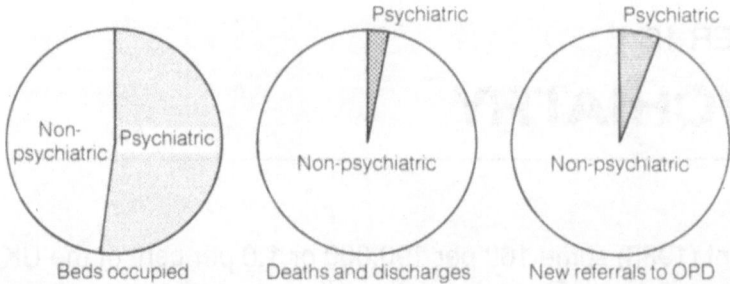

Figure 1   Hospital psychiatric resources per 100,000 (England, 1980) and percentages of total services (Health and Personal Social Services Statistics, 1982, Table 4.4)

Psychiatric inpatients

The numbers of patients occupying beds in psychiatric units in England have been falling year by year (Figure 2 and Table 2) from 189,000 in 1959 to 119,000 in 1980. The falls have been proportionately greater in those with mental illness than those mentally handicapped.

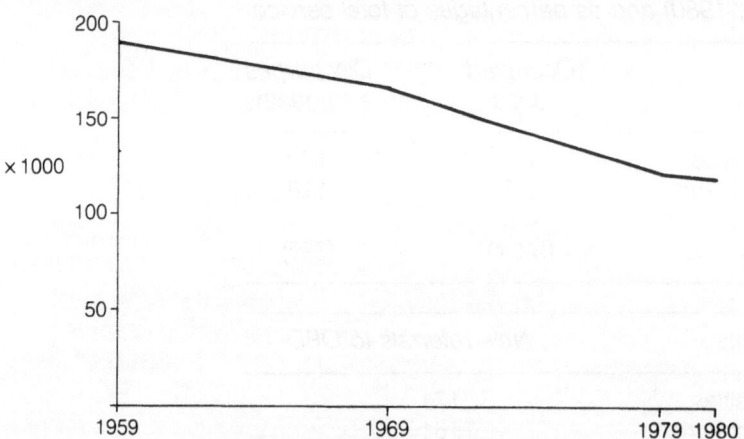

Figure 2   Psychiatric disorders (England): average numbers of beds occupied each year (to nearest thousand) (Health and Personal Social Services Statistics, 1982, Table 9.1)

164   PSYCHIATRY

Table 2   Psychiatric disorders (England): average number of beds occupied each year (to nearest thousand)

Average beds occupied in England	1959	1969	1979	1980
Mental illness	135,000	110,000	77,000	75,000
Mental handicap	54,000	56,000	45,000	44,000
Total	189,000	166,000	122,000	119,000

Source: *Health and Personal Social Services Statistics*, 1982, Table 9.1

Psychiatric deaths and discharges

The numbers of persons leaving psychiatric hospitals have been
increasing because of national policies and changing therapeutic
methods (Figure 3 and Table 3).

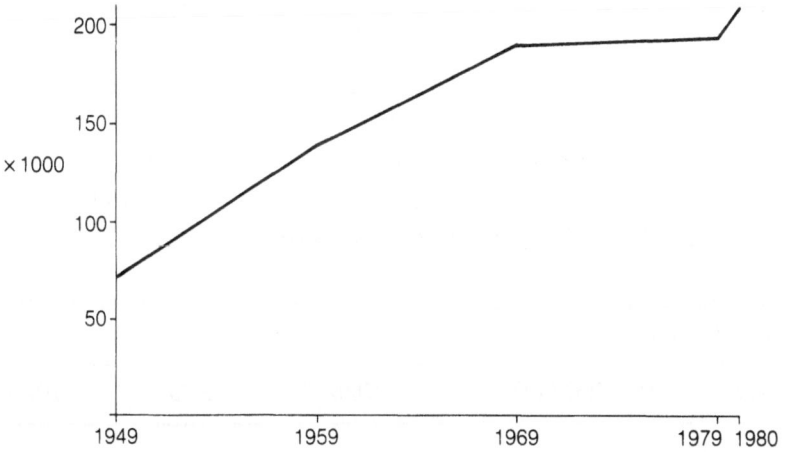

*Figure 3   Psychiatric disorders (England): discharges and deaths
from psychiatric hospitals (to nearest thousand)* (Health and
Personal Social Services Statistics, *1982, Table 9.1)*

Table 3   Psychiatric disorders (England): discharges and deaths per year
from psychiatric hospitals (to nearest thousand)

1949	1959	1969	1979	1980
72,000	139,000	190,000	194,000	209,000

Figures 2 and 3 and Tables 2 and 3 illustrate the increased utilization of psychiatric beds. With progressive reductions in numbers of available beds there will have been marked increases in numbers of persons leaving (passing through) these beds.

Admissions to psychiatric hospitals

'Admission' means entry or re-entry to a psychiatric hospital. There is a distinction between first admission of persons never previously admitted and those who are being readmitted.

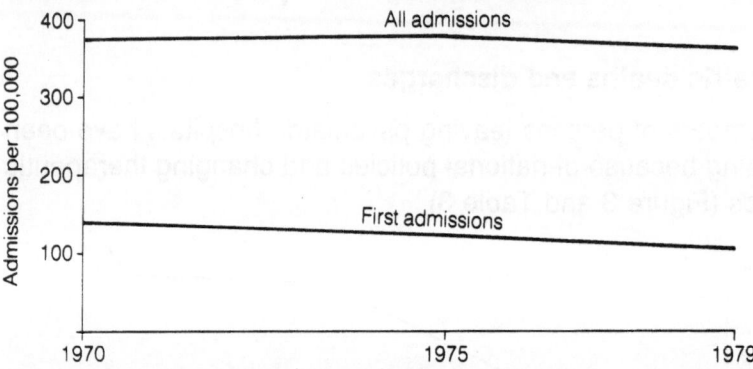

Figure 4   Admissions to psychiatric hospitals in England for all admissions and for first admissions (Health and Personal Social Services Statistics, *1982, Tables 9.2 and 9.3*)

Table 4   Admission to psychiatric hospitals in England, for all admissions and for first admissions

Admission rates per 100,000	1970	1975	1979
All admissions			
Males	313	314	301
Females	432	437	425
Total	374	377	365
First admissions	137	124	106
First admissions as percentage of all admissions	36%	33%	29%

Source: *Health and Personal Social Services Statistics*, 1982, Tables 9.2 and 9.3

Figure 4 and Table 4 show the rates per 100,000 for all admissions and for first admissions in 1970, 1975 and 1979. The rates for all admissions have been declining and so have the rates and proportions of first admissions. In 1970, first admissions were 36 per cent of all admissions and by 1979 the proportion had gone down to 29 per cent. The admission rates are always higher in females.

Age distribution

The ages of those admitted to psychiatric hospitals in rates per 100,000 in Table 5 show a steady and progressive rise with age. The percentage of first admissions out of all admissions is highest in the young (under 20) and in the very old.

Table 5   Admissions to psychiatric hospital (England, 1979)

	Under 10	10–	15–	20–	25–	35–	45–	55–	65–	75+	All ages
All psychiatric admissions in rates per 100,000	11	33	156	355	457	497	474	447	516	844	365
First admissions as percentage of all admissions	64%	67%	50%	35%	28%	24%	22%	23%	29%	41%	29%

New psychiatric outpatient referrals

Whilst admissions to psychiatric hospitals have been going down, new referrals to psychiatric outpatients departments have risen. Total attendances have increased more steeply because of greater number of attendances per patient referred (Figure 5 and Table 6).

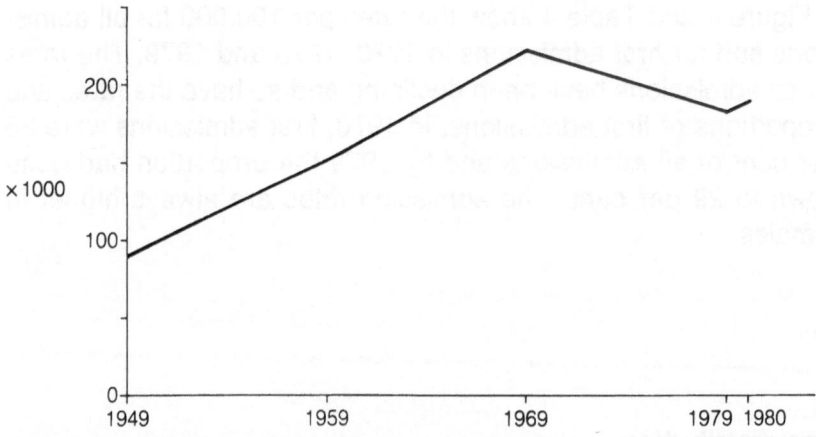

Figure 5   New referrals to psychiatric outpatient departments (England) (to nearest thousand) (Health and Personal Social Services Statistics, *1982, Table 9.1)*

Table 6   New referrals to psychiatric outpatient departments (England) to nearest thousand

Outpatient referrals and attendances	1949	1959	1969	1979	1980
New referrals	90,000	151,000	221,000	183,000	188,000
Total attendances	439,000	1,108,000	1,487,000	1,638,000	1,710,000
Mean number of attendances per new referral	4.9	7.3	6.7	9.0	9.1

Source: *Health and Personal Social Services Statistics,* 1982, Table 9.1

Psychiatric hospital admissions – by diagnosis

The diagnostic labels attached to those admitted to psychiatric hospitals in England in 1979 are shown in Figure 6 and Table 7. In order, schizophrenia, depression, psychoneurosis, alcoholism and senile dementia account for more than one-half but 'other' is the largest category.

Females outnumbered males by 2:1 for admissions, with some exceptions. The sex distribution was the same in both sexes in schizophrenia and males were predominant by 2:1 in alcoholism and in drug-dependence disorders.

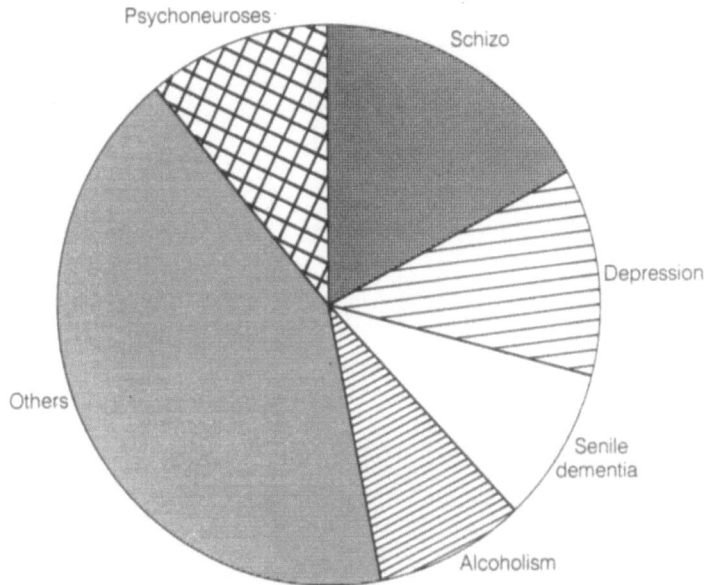

Figure 6 Psychiatric admissions by diagnosis (1979) (Health and Personal Social Services Statistics, *1982, Table 9.4)*

Table 7   Percentage psychiatric admissions by diagnosis (1979)

Diagnosis (%)									
Schizophrenia	Depression	Senile dementia	Other psychoses	Psycho neurosis	Alcoholism	Drug dependence	Personality behaviour	Others	Numbers
17	12	9	7	11	9	0.7	8	26	169,000

Source: *Health and Personal Social Services Statistics*, 1982, Table 9.4

Psychiatric patients' lengths of stay

In spite of the increasing annual numbers of persons in psychiatric hospitals who are discharged from hospital, the proportions who have been inpatients for long periods still are high, and are not changing very much.

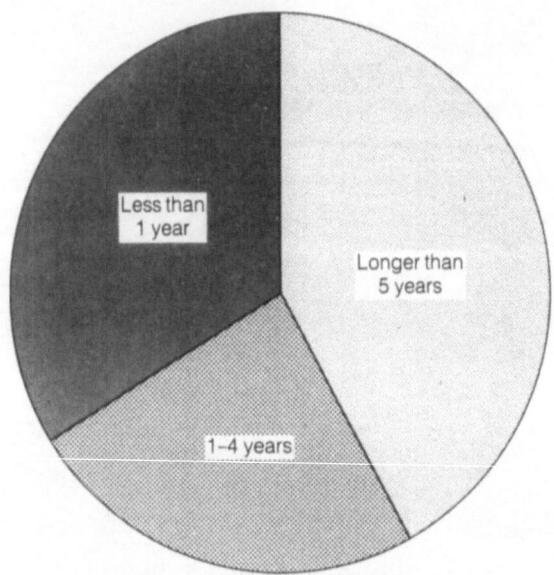

Figure 7 Psychiatric hospitals: lengths of stay of inpatients (Health and Personal Social Services Statistics, *1982, Table 9.5)*

Table 8 Psychiatric hospitals: lengths of stay of inpatients (percentages)

	1977	1979
Longer than 1 year		
Males	70	68
Females	65	64
Total	67	66
Longer than 5 years		
Males	51	48
Females	41	38
Total	45	42

In Figure 7 and Table 8 the percentages who have been in psychiatric hospital for longer than 1 year, and for longer than 5 years, have not changed greatly from 1977 to 1979. Two-thirds of all patients in psychiatric hospitals have been there longer than a year. Over 40 per cent have been in hospital for longer than 5 years.

It is of considerable interest that there are more males than females in these long-stay groups – whereas for most other indices of mental illness females outnumber males by 2:1.

Psychiatric patients leaving hospital – lengths of stay

Analysed in another way the lengths of stay of those patients leaving psychiatric hospitals (Figure 8 and Table 9) confirm that it

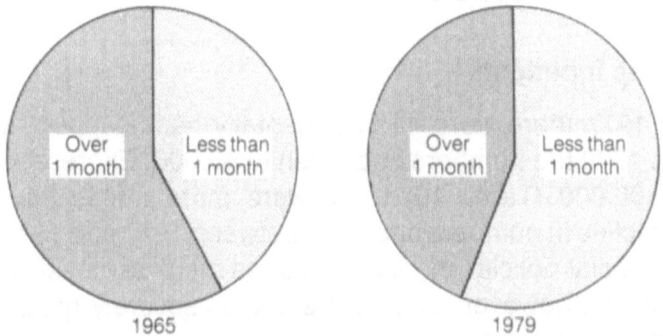

Figure 8   Patients leaving psychiatric hospitals: lengths of stay (Health and Personal Social Services Statistics, *1982, Table 9.6)*

Table 9   Patients leaving psychiatric hospitals: lengths of stay (percentage)

Lengths of stay	1965	1979
Less than 1 month	42	56
1–3 months	35	28
3 months–1 year	13	10
1–2 years	3	2
2–5 years	3	2
Over 5 years	4	2

Source: *Hospital and Personal Social Services Statistics*, 1982, Table 9.6)

is the very short-stay patients, who are in hospital for less than a month, that make up the largest proportion of the outflow. Very few of the 5-year + inpatients are discharged into the community and the percentages have gone down from 1965 to 1979.

The trends during this period show that whereas the percentage of short-stay (less than 1 month) inpatients has gone up from 42 to 56 per cent, for all longer stays the proportion has decreased.

MENTAL HANDICAP

Mental handicap is distinct from mental illness, and data related to it should be examined separately.

Mental handicap inpatients

In England in 1977 there were 48,000 mentally handicapped in hospital and in 1979 the numbers had fallen to 45,000. Expressed in rates per 100,000 (Table 10) there were more males than females. The decline in numbers and rates between 1977 and 1979 was due to the social policies of discharging as many as possible into the community; however, there are some so severely handicapped that they cannot be discharged.

Table 10   Mentally handicapped in hospitals

Rates per 100,000	1977	1979
Males	117	111
Females	90	85
Total	103	98
Numbers	48,000	45,000

Mentally handicapped – admissions

Paradoxically the admissions for mental handicapped have increased, whereas rates for inpatients have decreased (Figure 9 and Table 11). There were more females than males.

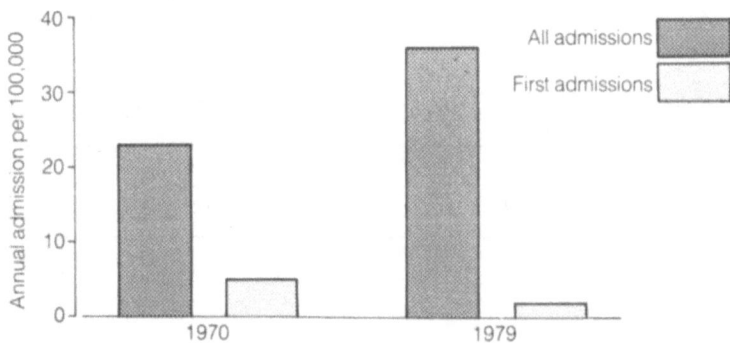

*Figure 9 Mental handicap: annual admissions 1970 and 1979 (England) in rates per 100,000 (*Health and Personal Social Services Statistics, *1982, Tables 9.7 and 9.8)*

Table 11   Mental handicap: annual admissions 1970 and 1979 (England)

Rates per 100,000	1970	1979
All admissions		
Male	27	41
Female	20	31
Total	23	36
First admissions	5	2
First admissions as percentage of all admissions	22%	6%

Source: *Health and Personal Social Services Statistics*, 1982, Tables 9.7 and 9.8

Thus, what is happening is that many of the same mentally handicapped are being admitted, discharged and readmitted.

Mental handicap – ages of admission

The ages of those admitted in 1979 (England) in rates per 100,000 are shown in Table 12. The trends are very different from those in mental illness (Figure 5 and Table 5), where the rates go up with age. In mental handicap the rates decline from the age of 20.

Table 12   Mental handicap: admissions (England, 1979) at different ages

Rates per 100,000	0–	10–	15–	20–	25–	35–	45–	55–	65+
All annual admissions	51	93	90	65	33	15	13	9	5

Mental handicap: reasons for admission

The most usual reasons for admission are 'social and other problems' and 'mental handicap' as a diagnosis (Figure 10 and Table 13)

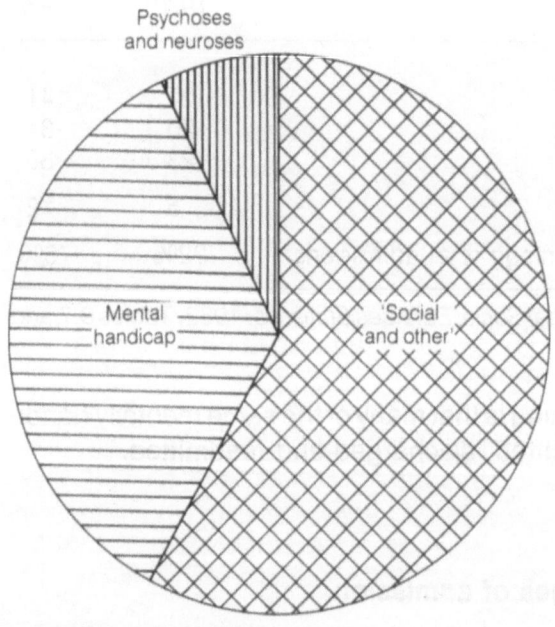

*Figure 10   Mental handicap: reasons for admission to hospital (England, 1979) (*Health and Personal Social Services Statistics, 1982, Table 9.9)

Table 13   Mental handicap: reasons for admission to hospital (England, 1979) (percentage)

Psychoses	Neuroses	Mental handicap	Social and other reasons
2	5	35	58

Mental handicap: length of stay

The great majority of mentally handicapped who are admitted to hospital are likely to stay there almost permanently (Figure 11 and Table 14). The proportion of those who have been in hospitals for longer than 5 years is increasing.

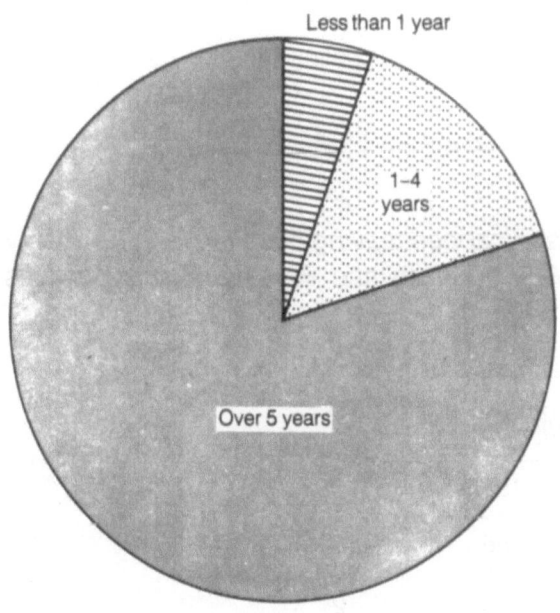

Figure 11   Mental handicap: length of stay in hospital (Health and Personal Social Services Statistics, *1982, Table 9.10*)

Table 14 Mental handicap: length of stay in hospital (percentages), England

	1977	1979
Longer than 1 year	94	95
Longer than 5 years	74	80

Source: *Health and Personal Social Services Statistics*, 1982, Table 9.10

Mentally handicapped leaving hospitals: lengths of stay

As with mental illness (Figure 8 and Table 9), of those mentally handicapped leaving hospitals the majority have been in for a very short time (less than 3 months) (Figure 12 and Table 15). After 3 months the chances of leaving in 1979 were less than in 1965.

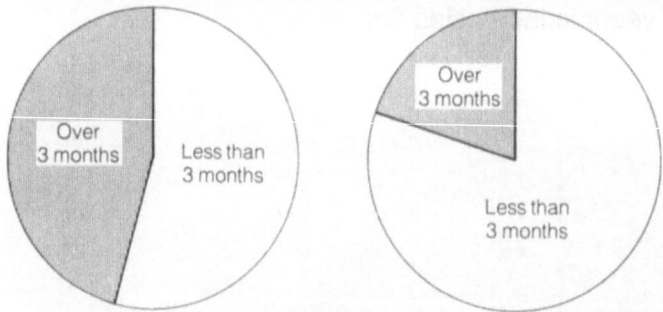

Figure 12   Mentally handicapped leaving hospital: lengths of stay (England, 1965 and 1979) (Health and Personal Social Services Statistics, *1982, Table 9.11)*

Table 15 Mentally handicapped leaving hospital: lengths of stay (percentages) (England, 1965 and 1979)

Lengths of stay	1965	1979
Less than 3 months	56	80
3 months–1 year	11	4
1–2 years	6	2
2–5 years	7	3
5 years +	20	11

COMMENTS

- Fifty-two per cent of all *hospital beds are for psychiatric disorders* (mental illness and mental handicap).
- *Occupied psychiatric beds* (for mental illness) were reduced by one-half from 1959 to 1980.
- Six per cent of all *new OPD referrals* are to psychiatric departments; but it is likely that one-quarter of referrals to general non-psychiatric clinics have a large emotional factor.
- *Discharges from psychiatric hospitals* trebled between 1949 and 1980 which, with fewer beds, indicates a faster throughput.
- Of *all psychiatric admissions* (in 1979) 29 per cent were first admissions and 71 per cent readmissions, suggesting that although more psychiatric patients are discharged into the community many will be readmitted.
- *Admissions to psychiatric hospitals* increase with age.
- *Psychiatric referrals to OPD* doubled from 1949 to 1980 and attendances quadrupled.
- *Diagnoses* as reasons for admission are in order:
  - schizophrenia;
  - depression;
  - psychoneurosis;
  - senile dementia;
  - alcoholism.
- In spite of increases in discharges and admissions there is a core of *long-stay patients* (in 1979):
  - 66 per cent had been inpatients for longer than 1 year;
  - 42 per cent had been inpatients for longer than 5 years.
- Most of those discharged from psychiatric hospitals are *short-stay cases* – 56 per cent had been in hospital for less than 1 month and 84 per cent less than 3 months.
- The situation in *mental handicap hospitals* is that 80 per cent have been inpatients for longer than 5 years and many of those discharged tend to be readmitted.
- The major change in policy has been to move *psychiatric patients back into the community*; with fewer psychiatric beds and more discharges. Those discharged are short-stay cases who come in and out and in again almost in rotation. There is

a core of severely disturbed persons who must have long-term custodial care. No tinkering with policies will really reduce the numbers.

● There are no fewer *psychiatric patients* overall, but more are being managed in the community and on an in/out admission pattern.

CHAPTER 13

MATERNITY SERVICES

Maternity services have changed in quality and quantity. Standards of care as shown in infant and maternal mortality rates have improved greatly. Birth rates have fallen markedly.

Birth rates

Birth rates fell to a low in 1977 and have risen since (Figure 1).

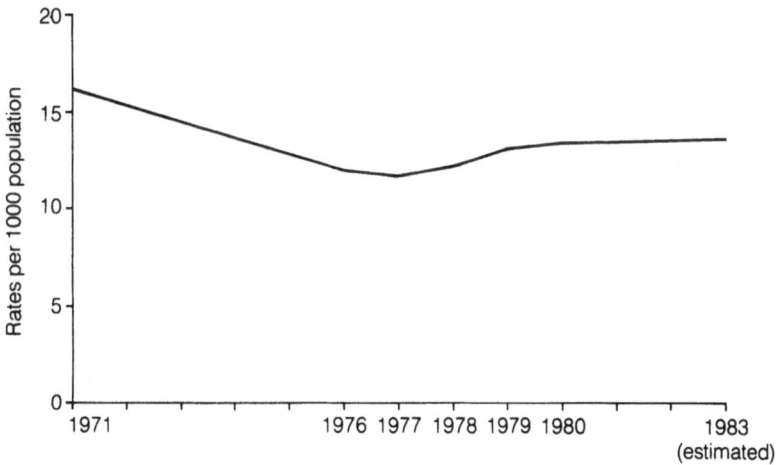

Figure 1 Total births 1949–1983 (1949–1971, England and Wales; 1971–1983 England) (Health and Personal Social Services Statistics, *1983, Table 1.1*)

Infant deaths

The rates of infant deaths are a recognized criterion of quality of maternity care and social standards. All the rates are put together in Figure 2, and all show marked reductions.

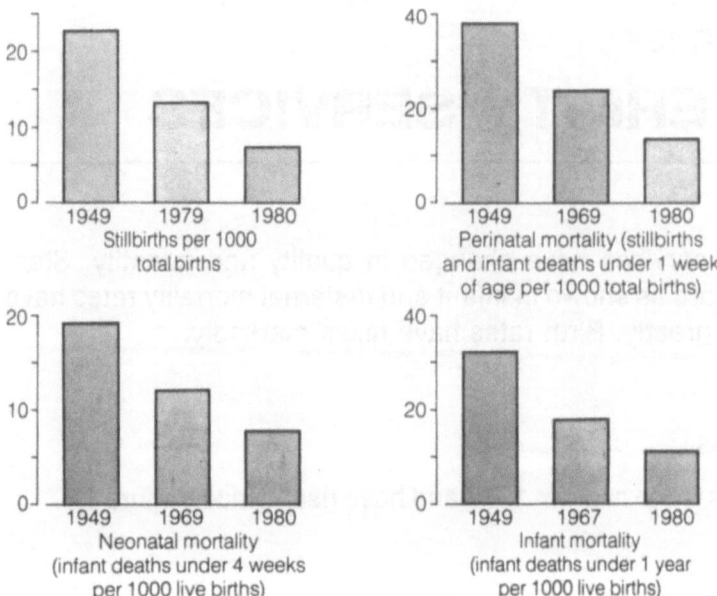

Figure 2   Infant deaths (1949–1980) (England and Wales, 1949–1971; England, 1971–1980) (Health and Personal Social Services *Statistics, 1982, Table 1.1)*

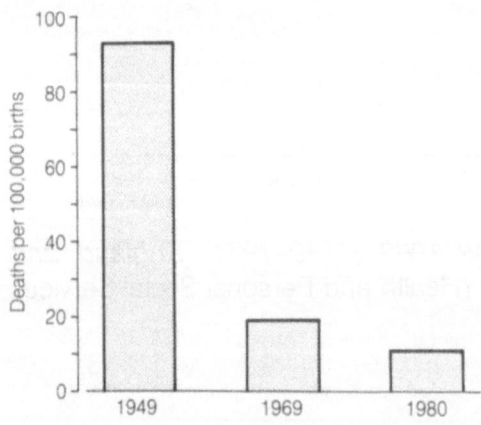

Figure 3   Maternal mortality (1949–1980) (1949–1971, England and Wales; 1971–1980, England) (Health and Personal Social Services Statistics, *1982, Table 1.1)*

Maternal mortality

Maternal mortality fell almost 10-fold from 1949, when 1 woman in every 1000 delivered died. In 1980 the rate was 1 per 10,000 (Figure 3).

There are differences in maternal mortality rates in the English regions. In 1976–1978 they ranged from 18.0 in N.E. Thames to 5.4 in Wessex.

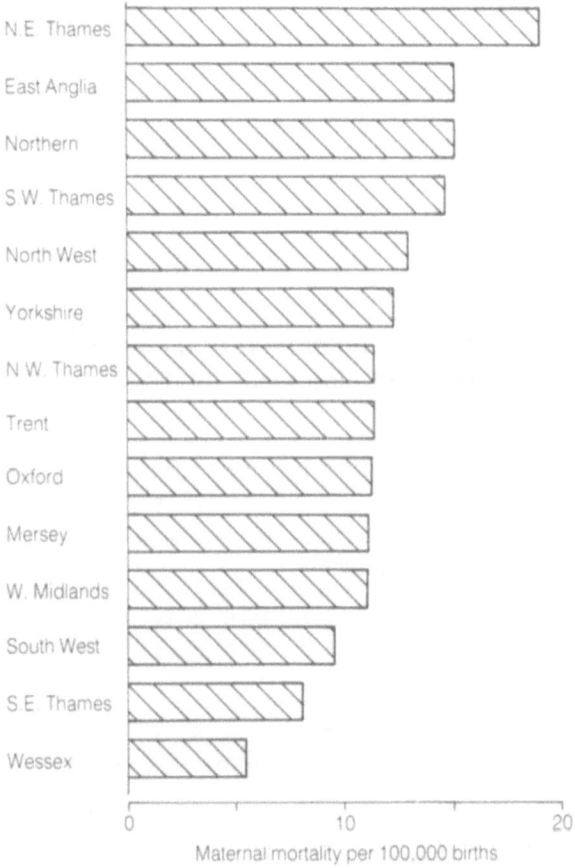

Figure 4   Maternal mortality rates per 100,000 total births (excluding abortions and anaesthetic deaths) by Regional Health Authority 1976–1978 (Cloake, E. (1982) Health Trends, *14, 106)*

Low birthweights of babies

Between 1971 and 1980 there was little difference in the proportions of low-birthweight babies. Since this is a risk factor for perinatal mortality it is surprising that the proportions did not fall – in fact there was a small rise from 6.3 to 6.8 per cent of all live births.

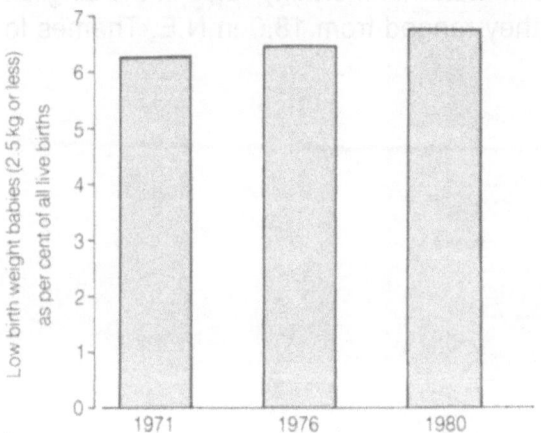

*Figure 5   Low-birthweight babies (percentage of all live births), England, 1971–1980 (*Health and Personal Social Services Statistics, *1982, Table 8.1)*

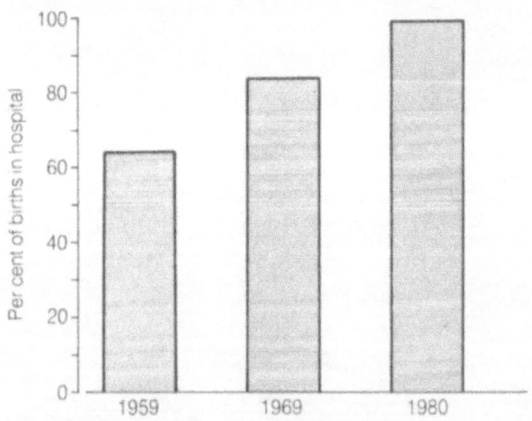

*Figure 6   Births in hospitals (England 1959–1980) (percentage of all births) (*Health and Personal Social Services Statistics, *1982, Table 8.1)*

Place of birth

Most births now take place in hospital. This was not always so. In 1959 one in three took place at home or in a nursing home (Figure 6).

General practitioner maternity beds

There has been a steady decline in the proportions of GP maternity beds in the NHS as a percentage of all obstetric beds (Figure 7).

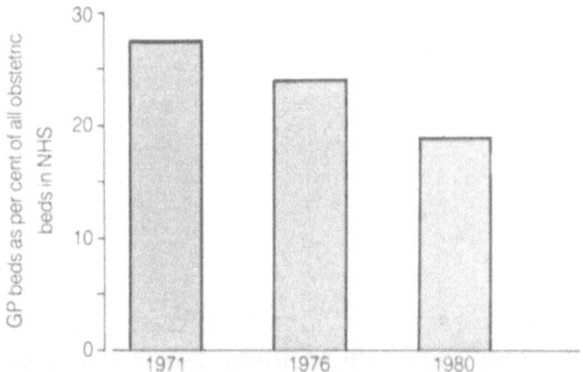

Figure 7   GP maternity beds as a percentage of all obstetric beds (England, 1971–1980) (Health and Personal Social Services Statistics, *1982, Table 8.1)*

Staffing

Total medical obstetric staff in England in NHS increased from 1806 in 1970 to 2313 in 1980, and of these consultants increased from 510 to 612.

Hospital midwives increased from 15,002 in 1974 to 17,163 in 1980.

Community midwives decreased from 4237 in 1974 to 2773 in 1980 – mainly because of fall in domiciliary deliveries.

Work of domiciliary midwives

The work of domiciliary midwives has changed. No longer does it consist of home deliveries or hospital deliveries, but rather of postnatal care of mothers discharged early from hospital (Figure 8). The total case-load per midwife in England appeared to be 222 cases.

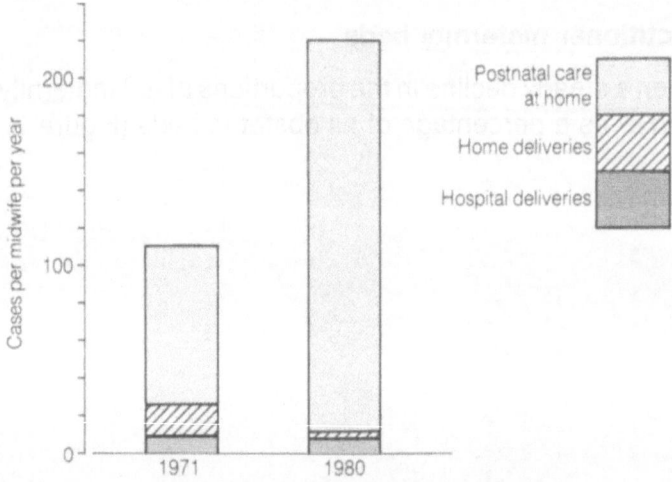

*Figure 8   Community midwives: annual numbers of cases of home deliveries, hospital deliveries and home postnatal care per midwife (England, 1971–1980) (*Health and Personal Social Services Statistics, *1982, Table 8.1)*

COMMENT

- *Birth rate* fell to a low of 11.7 per 1000 in 1977 from 17.1 in 1949, and is now 13.6.
- *Infant and maternal mortalities* continue to decline but still there are regional inequalities.
- Ninety-nine per cent of *all deliveries* are in NHS hospitals.
- On average a community midwife can expect no more than three *home deliveries* in a year, and a GP once every 6–7 years.
- It is likely that up to 20 per cent of deliveries take place in *GP maternity hospital beds*.

CHAPTER 14

EYES AND TEETH

COMMUNITY OPHTHALMIC SERVICES

There are three groups involved in eye testing and prescribing spectacles in the NHS:

- ophthalmic medical practitioners;
- ophthalmic opticians;
- dispensing opticians.

Ophthalmic medical practitioners test vision and prescribe for spectacles; ophthalmic opticians test vision and supply the spectacles; and dispensing opticians dispense and supply the spectacles on prescriptions of medical practitioners.

Figure 1 and Table 1 show that the total number of these three groups in 1980 was 7636, a modest increase of 15 per cent over 1969. There was a fall in the numbers of ophthalmic medical practitioners, no real change in ophthalmic opticians but a doubling of dispensing opticians.

Table 1   NHS opticians and ophthalmic medical practitioners (1969 and 1982) (England)

	1969	1980	Percentage change
Ophthalmic medical practitioners	853	837 (11%)	− 2
Ophthalmic opticians	4654	4715 (63%)	+ 1
Dispensing opticians	1104	2084 (26%)	+ 90
Total	6611	7636 (100%)	+ 15

Source: Health and Personal Social Services Statistics, 1982, Table 5.6

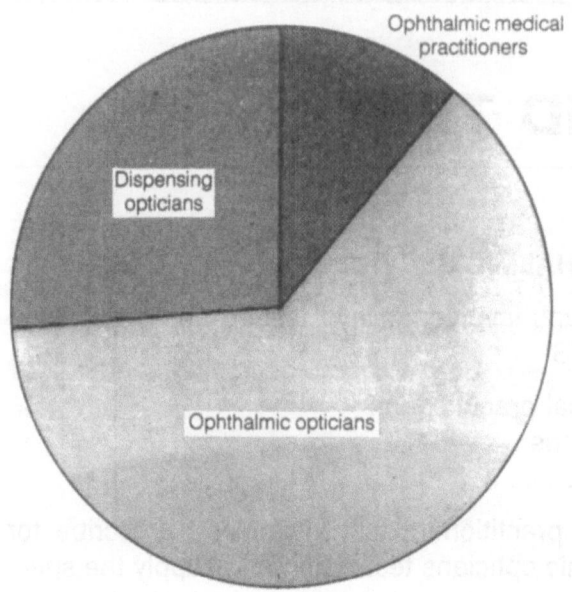

Figure 1   NHS opticians and ophthalmic medical practitioners (1969 and 1980) (England) (Health and Personal Social Services Statistics, *1982, Table 5.6*)

Sight tests

The number of eye tests in England in 1980 was 8.4 million, and in 1969 it was 6.4 million. In 1980 this was a rate of 170 per 1000

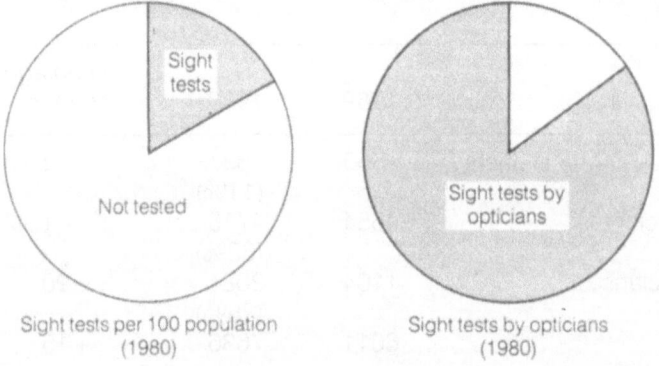

Sight tests per 100 population
(1980)

Sight tests by opticians
(1980)

Figure 2   NHS sight tests (1969 and 1980) (England) (Health and Personal Social Services Statistics, *1982, Table 5.6*)

of the population. It is likely that over one-third of the population have spectacles.

Most of the sight tests are carried out by opticians (85 per cent in 1980). Of all sight tests, in 75 per cent spectacles were prescribed (Figure 2 and Table 2).

Table 2   NHS sight tests (1969 and 1980) (England)

	1969	1980	Percentage change
Total number of sight tests	6.4 million	8.4 million	
Rate per 1000	146	170	+21
Percentage carried out by ophthalmic opticians	80	85	+6
Percentage of sight tests in which spectacles were prescribed	75	75	—

Source: Health and Personal Social Services Statistics, 1982, Table 5.6

Frames supplied

After a sight test if spectacles are prescribed (and they are in 75 per cent) the patient has a choice of NHS frames (cheap), private frames (expensive) or the old frame may be reglazed. In Figure 3 and Table 3, it is evident that in adults there is an equal distribution between private and NHS frames. In children the majority have NHS frames.

Table 3 NHS spectacle frames supplied, 1981 (percentages) (England)

	Adults	Children
NHS frames	35	76
Private frames	39	12
Existing frame reglazed	26	12

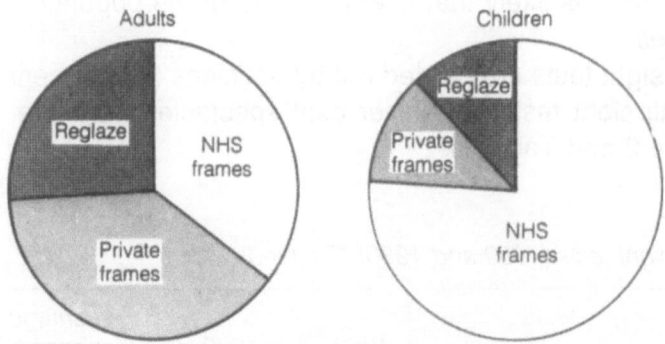

Figure 3 NHS spectacle frames supplied, 1981 (percentages) (England) (Health and Personal Social Services Statistics, *1982, Table 5.6*)

COMMUNITY DENTAL SERVICES

General dental practitioners (dentists)

There are approximately half as many dentists in England as general medical practitioners (Figure 4 and Table 4). The numbers are increasing and therefore the number of persons per dentist is

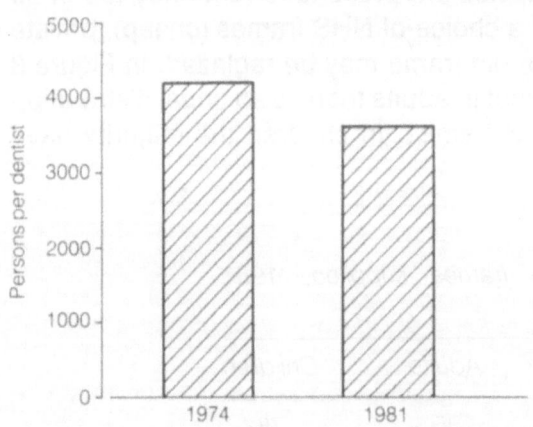

Figure 4 Persons per dentist (1981) (England) (Health and Personal Social Services Statistics, *1982, Table 3.2a*)

188   EYES AND TEETH

going down. There is unequal distribution in England. In the N.W. Thames region in 1981 there was one dentist to 2379 persons, and in the Northern region one to 5002.

Table 4   Numbers of dentists and persons per dentist (1981) (England)

	1974	1981	Percentage change
Numbers of dentists	11,023	12,835	+ 14
Persons per dentist	4195	3603	– 14

Source: *Health and Personal Social Services Statistics*, 1982, Table 3.2a

Dental treatment

The total services given by dentists under NHS quadrupled between 1949 and 1981 and the cost increased by over 100-fold (not allowing for inflation) (Figure 5 and Table 5). In 1981 the NHS payments to dentists averaged at £22,000 per dentist – most have other incomes from private work.

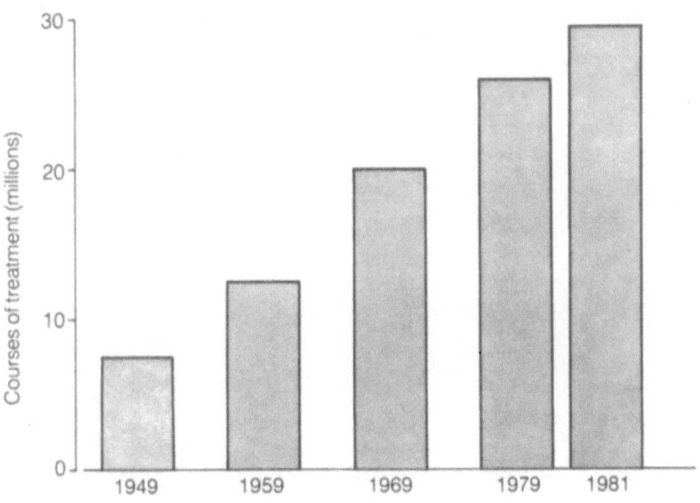

Figure 5   NHS dental treatment (1949–1981) (England) (Health and Personal Social Services Statistics, *1982, Tables 5.1 and 5.4)*

Table 5   NHS dental treatment and costs (1949–1981) (England)

	1949	1959	1969	1979	1981
Total courses of treatment (million)	7.5	12.5	20	27	29
Payments to dentists (£ million)	41	48	62	240	455
Payment to each dentist	£5100	—	—	—	£22,000

Source: *Health and Personal Social Services Statistics*, 1982, Tables 5.1 and 5.4

Costs

For 1981 the costs for the 29 million treatments represented:

- number of courses per 1000 persons   628
- average cost per course   £15.66
- cost per person in population   £10 (approx.)

Dental care by age

Most dental care is provided for children and young adults (Figure 6 and Table 6).

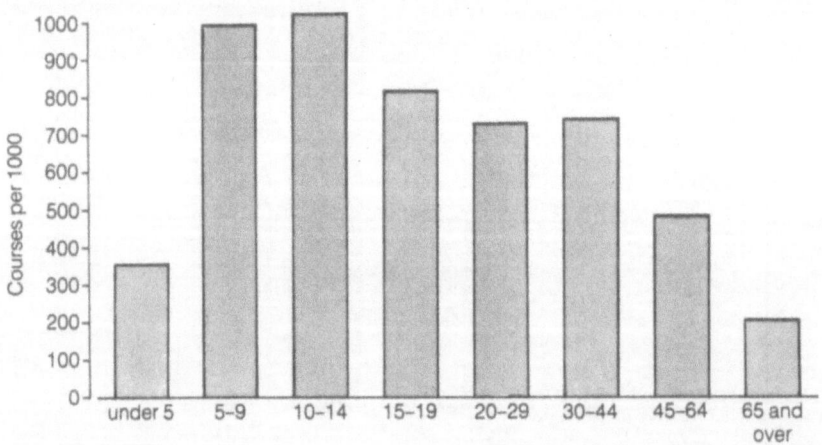

Figure 6   Dental care by age (Health and Personal Social Services Statistics, *1982, Table 5.4)*

190   EYES AND TEETH

Table 6 Dental care by age (courses per 1000)

0–	5–	10–	15–	20–	30–	45–	65+	All
355	995	1022	816	730	742	482	204	628

Source: *Health and Personal Social Services Statistics*, 1982, Table 5.4

Care for mothers and children

In addition to independent general dental practitioners (12,835 in 1981) there were 1749 dentists employed by local authorities to provide care for schoolchildren, infants (pre-school) and expectant mothers. They inspected 5.4 million cases in 1981, of whom 45 per cent needed treatment. The school dental service was the largest sector:

- 5.3 million cases examined (63 per cent of school population)
- 2.3 million (43 per cent) needed treatment
- 1.2 million (23 per cent) received treatment

(Data from *Health and Personal Social Services Statistics*, 1982, Tables 6.9–6.12.)

COMMENTS

- One-third of the population wear *spectacles*.
- Eighty-five per cent of eye tests are by *opticians*.
- *Spectacles* are prescribed in 75 per cent of tests.
- *New NHS frames* are supplied to 36 per cent of adults and 76 per cent of children requiring spectacles.
- Numbers of *general dental practitioners* (GDP) increased by 14 per cent, 1974–1981.
- There is one GDP to 3603 persons, but there are gross regional variations.
- Most *dental care* is given to children age 5–15.
- These eye and dental services are under Family Practitioner Committees, but opticians and GDPs are *independent contractors*.

CHAPTER 15

SCHOOL MEDICAL SERVICE

The need for special health services for children in school is being questioned. The staff of the school medical service comprises many more nurses than health visitors and doctors (Figure 1) (Nurses: 2671; doctors and health visitors: 1827). In 1977 a study of the school nursing and medical services in the north Paddington district of London revealed that over one-third of children had problems (Figure 3). The proportions were higher in infant school (5–7) than in junior school (8–9). The types of problems were more physical than behavioural (Table 1).

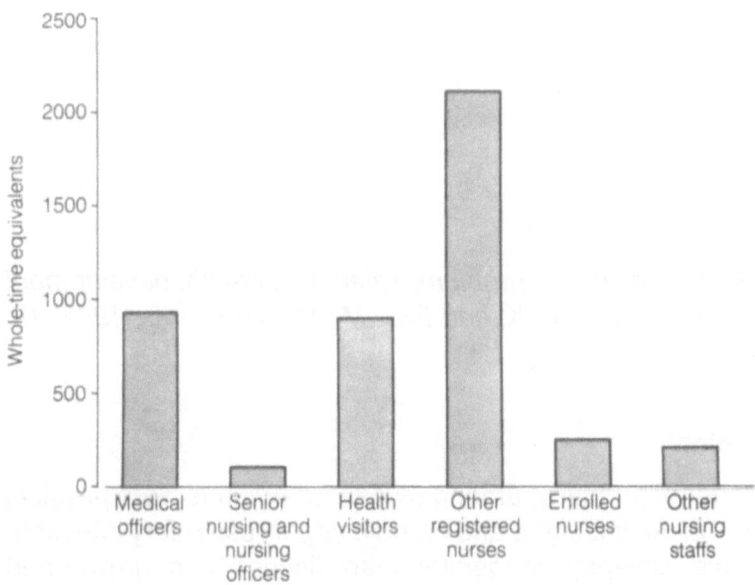

*Figure 1   Staff, school medical service, England, 1979 (*Health and Personal Social Service Statistics, *1982, Table 6.3)*

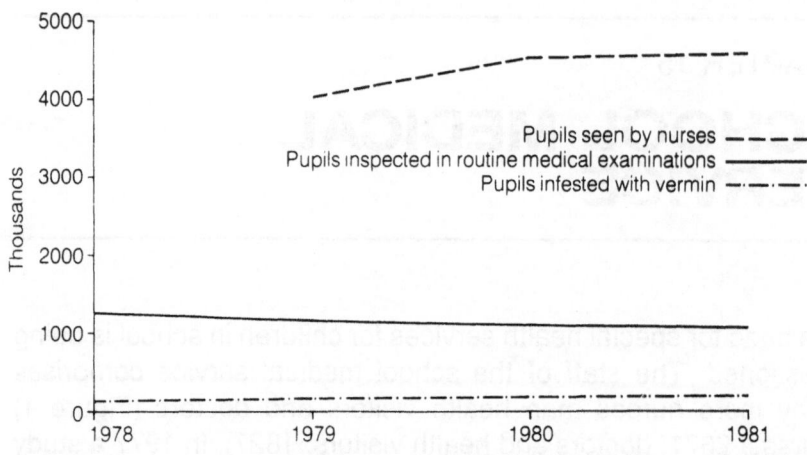

Figure 2 School children, health surveillance, England, 1978–1981 (Health and Personal Social Services Statistics, *1982, Table 6.4)*

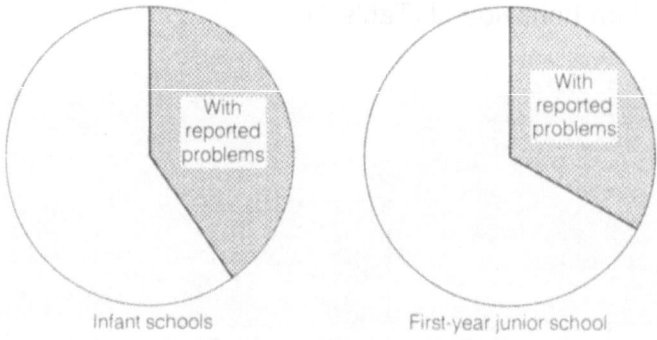

Infant schools   First-year junior school

Figure 3 Prevalence of problems relating to health, development or behaviour (Whitmore, K. and Bax, M., Health Trends, *1984, 14, p. 52)*

The problems

One-quarter of problems among 5-year-old entrants were physical disorders, including acute and chronic upper respiratory infection, otitis media, epilepsy, congenital heart disease, poor growth and obesity, and a variety of skin diseases; another quarter were reduced visual acuity and hearing. Two per cent had marked errors of articulation and 8 per cent were significantly retarded in

Table 1   Type of problems identified

| | Percentage of children with problems | |
	351 entrants to infant school	325 first-year juniors
Physical	15	20
Visual	8	9
Hearing	7	1
Speech and language	8	1
Behaviour including enuresis	9	3
Cognitive	14	5

Source: Whitmore. K. and Bax, M., *Health Trends*, 1982, 14, p. 52)

language development. Behavioural problems included feeding and sleep disturbances, soiling and enuresis, temper tantrums, over-activity, clumsiness and stealing. Among the 7-year-old juniors physical problems (including defects of vision and speech) predominated.

Prior knowledge

Only half the children with confirmed problems on entry to school had been seen in child health clinics before; only 6 per cent of children with problems on entry to school had attended their family doctor during the previous 12 months because of these problems.

Management

Management involved observation, treatment, referral and advice to parents and teachers. Half the problems were referred by school doctors (to GPs or specialists) and half were managed by the school doctors themselves.

Outcome

Half the problems among entrants and first-year juniors had resolved within 12–18 months and another quarter had been reduced. Four per cent of parents did not follow the school doctor's advice to take the child to the family doctor or to see a hospital specialist. In an effective school health service, six principles involve children, parents and teachers (Figure 4).

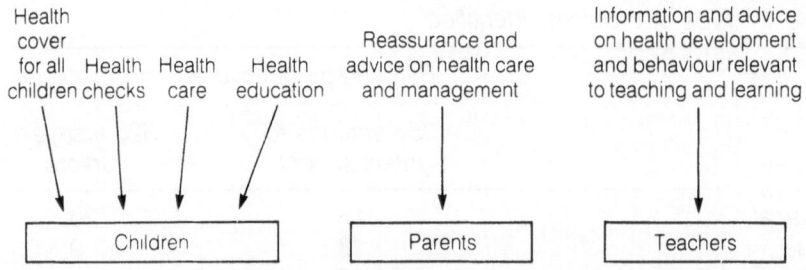

Figure 4   Six principal objectives of the school health services

COMMENT

- Within a national health system that includes general practitioners who are responsible for the care of children registered with them, it is difficult to fit the school medical service into an important niche.
- Yet it acts to provide general preventive care to pick up conditions that have been missed and are in need of treatment and more especially to assist teachers in defining problems that hinder normal educational development. It has to be asked: who should carry out this work – school medical service or general practitioners?

CHAPTER 16

QUALITY AND OUTCOMES

The structure and processes of medical and health care have to be related to the outcomes of such care. There has to be critical evaluation of benefits, if any, of such care.

In a National Health Service it should, in theory, be possible to examine and assess trends and results of care provided. Efficiency, effectiveness and economics have to be based on such evaluations and assessments. Sadly, there is no good recognizable system in the British NHS that collects and evaluates data in quality and outcomes on which policies can be made and implemented. In this sections we present piecemeal data to demonstrate possibilities of data analysis and deficiencies in data available.

Prevention

Prevention is a great concept. No-one questions that prevention of premature death, disease and suffering must be promoted. There have been some definable procedures aimed at preventing disease and avoiding social suffering. Four are examined: cervical cytology, immunization, care of expectant mothers, and family planning and legal abortion.

CERVICAL CYTOLOGY

In 1980 approximately one-quarter of women between 15 and 50 had cervical cytology carried out, compared with 20 per cent in 1973 (Figure 1 and Table 1). The policy in Britain is for repeat examination in 5 years when the results are normal, and more frequently in certain age groups (under 20) and when some minor abnormality exists. There are no data on the proportion of women having cytological examination in 5-year periods. In the 15–50 age group it is likely to be over 60 per cent.

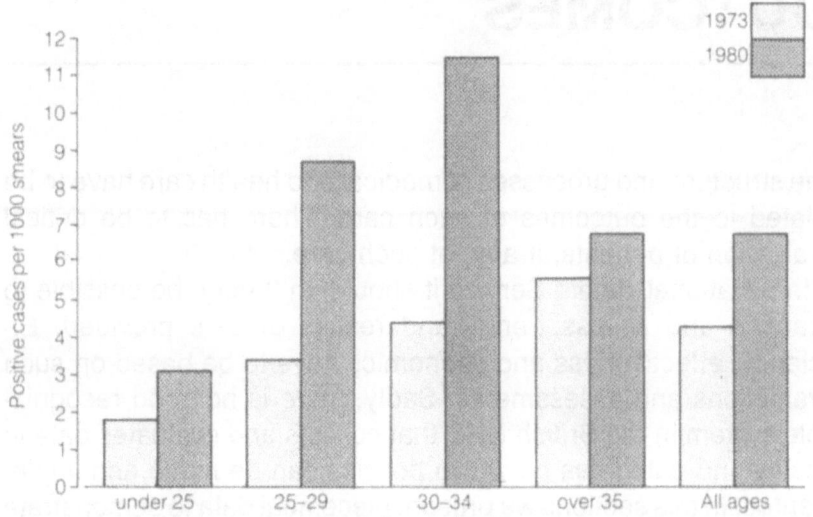

Figure 1 Cervical cytology examination (England) 1973 and 1980 – numbers of positive smears per 1000 (Health and Personal Social Services Statistics, *1982, Table 10.2*)

Table 1   Cervical cytology examination, England, 1937 and 1980

Age	Smears examined (thousands)		Positive cases per 1000 smears examined	
	1973	1980	1973	1980
All ages	2226	2789	4.3	6.8
(Percentage of women aged 15–50)	(20%)	(25%)		
Under 25	452	671	1.8	3.1
25–29	435	444	3.4	8.7
30–34	316	384	4.4	11.5
Over 35	1023	1291	5.6	6.8

Source: *Health and Personal Social Services Statistics,* 1982, Table 10.2

The effects on the incidence (registrations), mortality and 5-year survival rates of cancer of the cervix cannot be fairly assessed because the smearing programme has not been going long enough. Table 2 (on data from *Trends in Cancer Survival in Great Britain* – Cancer Research Campaign (CRC), London, 1982) shows some improvements in registration and mortality rates. The 5-year survival rate for invasive cervical cancer in England and Wales in 1973 was 54 per cent (see also page 221). It may be that more recent data will show greater benefits.

Table 2 Cancer of cervix: trends in incidence and mortality rates (per 100,000 population)

Registration (incidence) per 100,000		Mortality per 100,000	
1966/1970	1971/1974	1961/1965	1976/1978
16.8	15.6	9.4	7.6

Source: CRC, 1982

Smears by source

Most of the increase since 1965 is due to the work of general practitioners. Between 1970 and 1980 the proportion of smears taken by general practitioners rose from 23 to 43 per cent (Figures 2 and 3).

Abnormal smears by age groups

Overall abnormalities are reported in 6.8 per 1000 smears. The highest rate was in 30–34 age group (Figure 1).

Abnormal smears by source

The abnormality rate is 6.8 per 1000. The highest rate is from hospital outpatient departments, because they have selected patients referred by GPs with likely abnormalities.

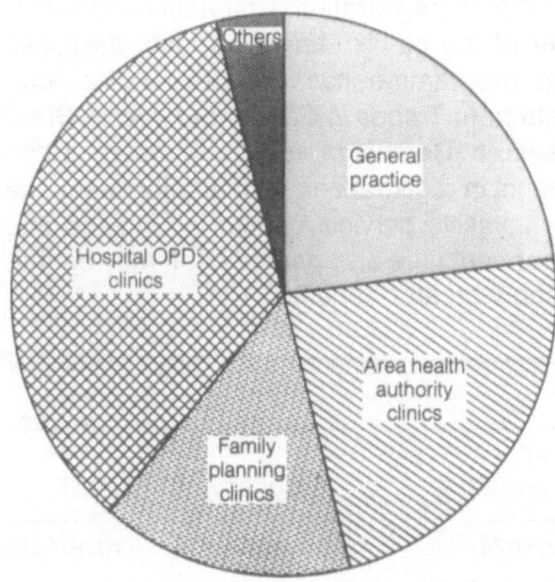

Figure 2   Smears by source, 1970, England and Wales (Roberts, A. (1982) Health Trends, *14, 41)*

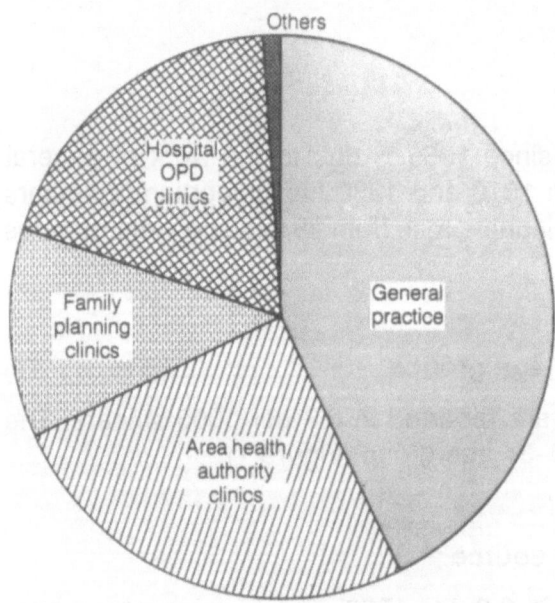

Figure 3   Smears by source, 1980, England and Wales (Roberts, A. (1982) Health Trends, *14, 41)*

Results of biopsies on abnormal smears

Figure 4 shows that confirmed cancer of cervix was found in 50 per cent of biopsies.

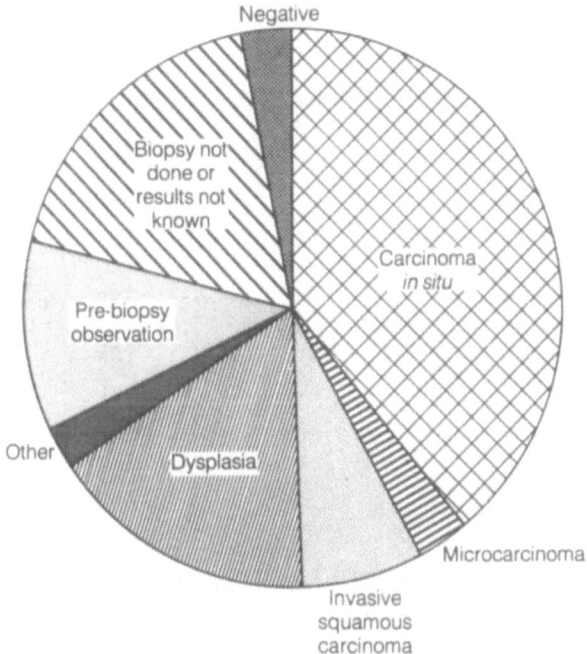

Figure 4   Biopsy results (based on all smears detected for the first time as positive in the first 3 months of each year) 1980 (Roberts, A. (1982) Health Trends, *14, 41)*

IMMUNIZATION

In Britain between 1969 and 1981, following anxiety over the possible side effects of pertussis vaccine, the acceptance rates for immunization against whooping cough were almost halved (Figure 5 and Table 3). The acceptance rates for other available vaccines increased or remained static.

Whereas the acceptance rates for immunization against diphtheria, tetanus, poliomyelitis, rubella and tuberculosis were over 70 per cent, those against measles, in 1981, were 55 per cent, and against whooping cough 45 per cent. The effects of the decline in acceptance rate for immunization against whooping cough show an increase in its notifications since the low rate of 1971 (Figure 6).

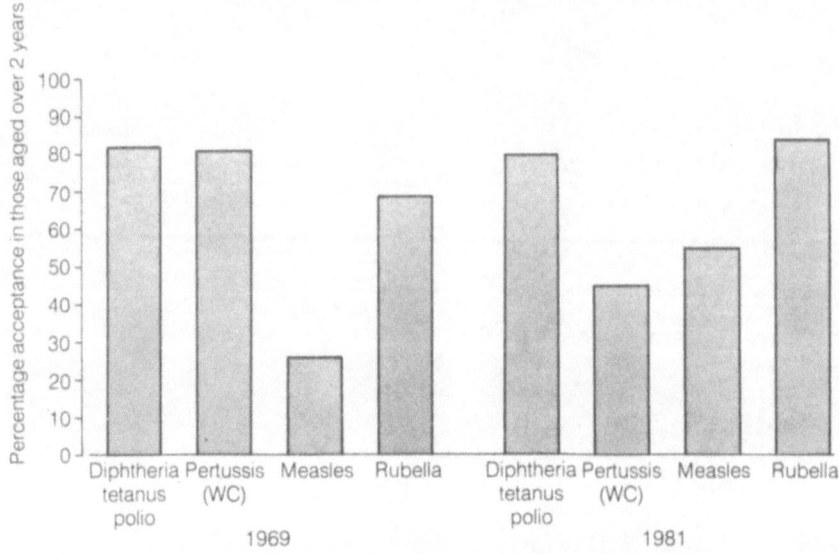

Figure 5   Acceptance rates for immunization in 1969 and 1981 (percentage of children, England) (Health and Personal Social Services Statistics, *1982, Table 10.1)*

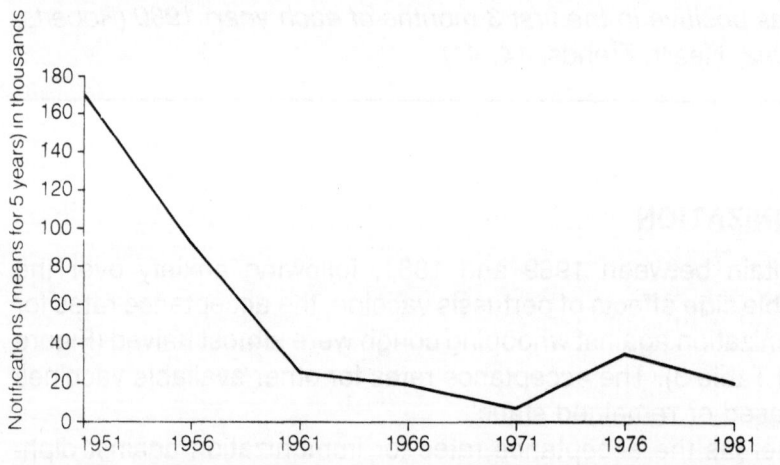

Figure 6   Mean quinquennial notifications of whooping cough in England (DHSS; personal data)

The immunization programme against whooping cough has been actively promoted since the early 1960s.

Table 3   Acceptance rates for immunization, 1969 and 1981

	Percentage acceptance rates		Percentage of children	
	1969		1981	
	Age under 1 year	Age over 2 years	Age under 1 year	Age over 2 years
Diphtheria	68	83	73	84
Tetanus	68	83	73	83
Pertussis (WC)	66	81	45	45
Poliomyelitis	65	80	72	72
Measles	—	26	—	55
Rubella	—	69 (1977)	—	84
Tuberculosis TB negative 'Negatives' immunized	—	87	—	90
with BCG	—	97	—	98

Source: *Health and Personal Social Services Statistics*, 1982, Table 10.1

MATERNAL AND PERINATAL MORTALITY
(see also Chapter 13)

Table 4   Maternal mortality and perinatal mortality rates, 1949–1979, England

	1949	1959	1969	1979
Maternal mortality (per 1000 births)	0.97	0.38	0.19	0.11
Perinatal mortality (per 1000 births) (all deaths under 1 week of age)	38.0	34.1	23.4	14.6

Source: *Health and Personal Social Services Statistics*, 1982, Table 1.1

Whether it be through better antenatal, intranatal and postnatal care, or because of improved social conditions, the maternal and perinatal mortality rates have continued to improve (Figure 7).

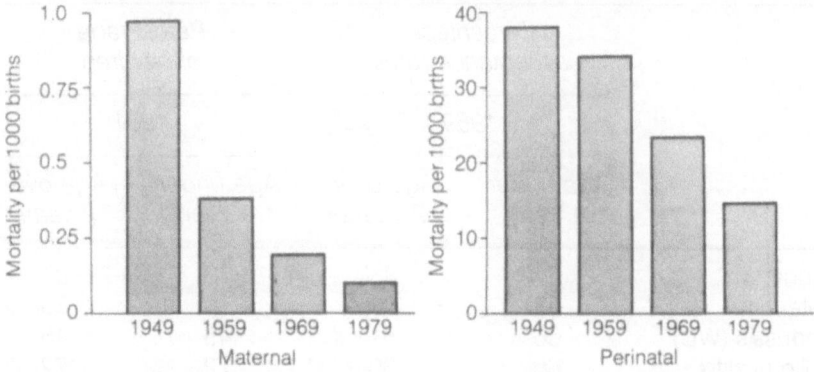

*Figure 7   Maternal mortality and perinatal mortality rates, 1949–1979, England (*Health and Personal Social Services Statistics, *1982, Table 1.1)*

FAMILY PLANNING (see also Chapter 13)

Since 1975 all family planning services have been provided free of charge in the NHS. A little more than one-third of all women age

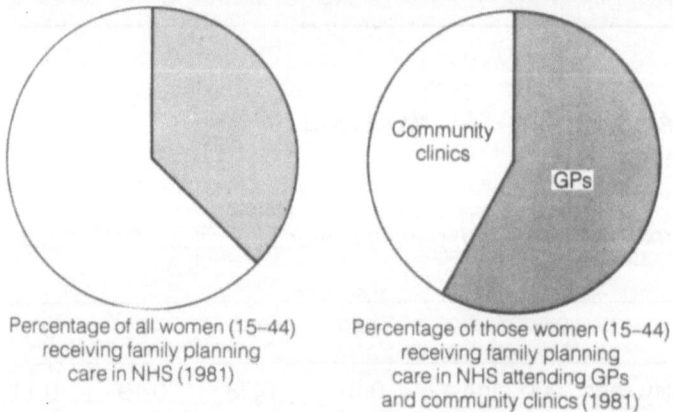

*Figure 8   Family planning services in NHS – persons attending clinics and GPs (*Health and Personal Social Services Statistics, *1982, Table 6.5)*

15–44 in England attended community clinics or their general practitioners for family planning advice. Of those attending in 1981, 58 per cent attended their general practitioners and in 1977 the proportion was 56 per cent. In 1977 the live birth rate was 11.6 per 1000 and in 1981 it was 13.4 per 1000 (Figure 8 and Table 5).

Table 5   Family planning services in NHS – persons attending

Thousands	1977	1981
Community clinics	1537 (44%)	1477 (42%)
General practitioners	2038 (56%)	2092 (58%)
Total	3575 (100%)	3569 (100%)
Percentage of women aged 15–44	39	37
Live births per 1000	11.6	13.4

Sources: Health and Personal Social Services Statistics, 1982, Table 6.5

FAMILY PLANNING SERVICES

Between 1977 and 1981 the number of patients seen at community

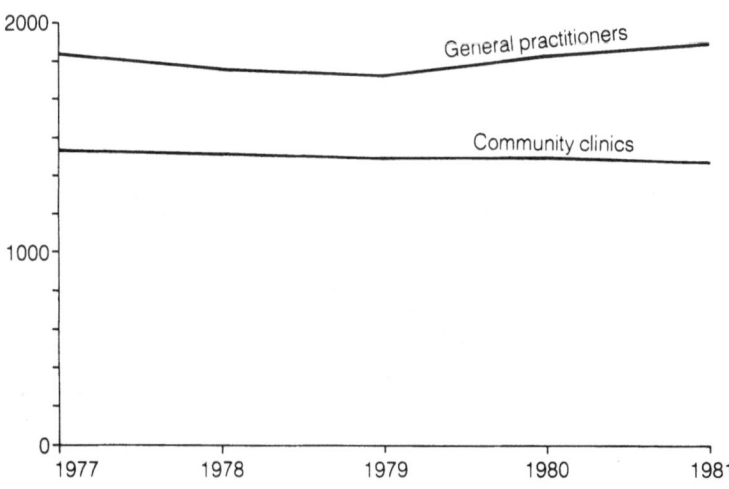

Figure 9   The number of patients seen by general practitioners and at community clinics 1977–1981, England (thousands) (Health and Personal Social Services Statistics, 1982, Table 6.5)

clinics declined slightly, whereas the number seen by general practitioners slightly increased after 1979 (Figure 9).

Contrary to common belief the use of reversible contraception by married women in the childbearing years or by their husbands appeared to decline between 1967 and 1975 (Figure 10) because of an increase in use of permanent (irreversible) methods such as sterilization.

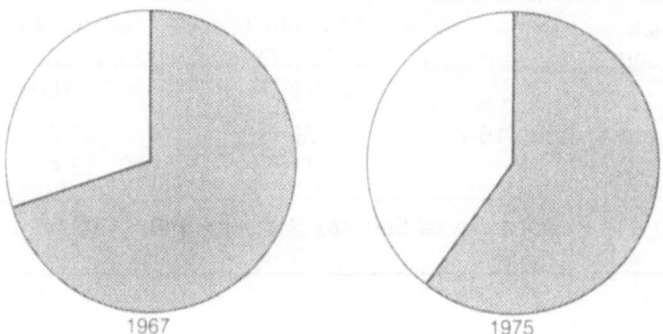

Figure 10   The proportion of married women or their husbands using reversible contraception, England and Wales (Bone, M. R. (1980) Health Trends, 12, 87)

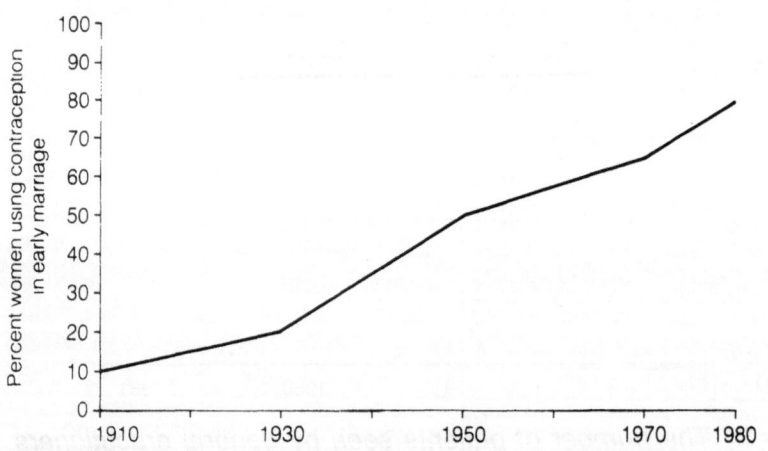

Figure 11   Women using contraception in early marriage (1910– 1980) (Bone, M.R. (1980) Health Trends, 12, 87)

Extent of use of contraception in earliest stage of marriage

The growth of use of contraception in early marriage (from marriage to first pregnancy) has increased from 10 per cent in 1910 to over 80 per cent in 1980 (Figure 11).

Methods of reversible contraception

The 'pill' has been growing in popularity (Table 6 and Figure 12). The sheath still is used by about one-quarter, and other specific methods are much less popular.

Table 6   Current use of contraception in 1970 and 1975 (percentage of married women 16–40 years using each method

Method	1970	1975
Pill	25 ⎤	42 ⎤
Condom	36 ⎬ 72	25 ⎬ 79
Diaphragm	6 ⎟	3 ⎟
IUD	5 ⎦	9 ⎦
Withdrawal	19	7
Safe period	6	1
Other	N/A	4
Abstinence/none	11	12

Source: Bone, M. R. (1980) *Health Trends*, **12**, 87

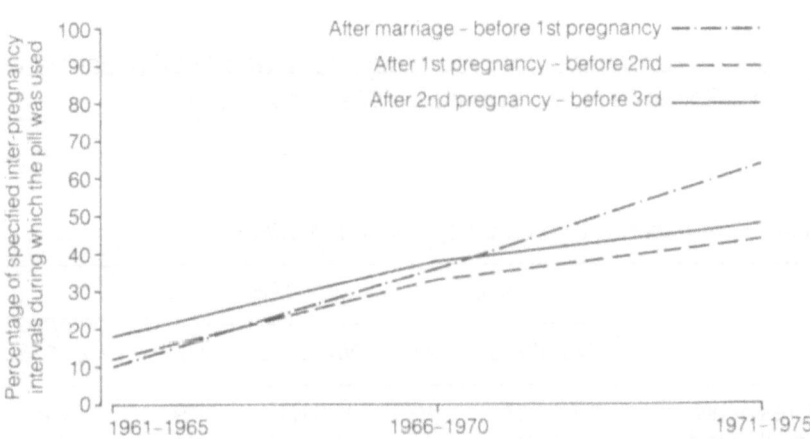

Figure 12   Growth in the use of the pill (Bone, M. R. (1980) Health Trends, *12, 87)*

TERMINATION OF PREGNANCY

In spite of the availability of free family planning services the numbers of terminations of pregnancy (in England) doubled from 1970 to 1980 (Figure 13 and Table 7). The rate of increase was 3-fold for women not resident in UK and 1.8-fold for UK residents. The proportions of non-UK residents of the total numbers were 13 per cent in 1970 and 21 per cent in 1980. For UK residents the rates per 1000 of women aged 15–44 were 7.7 in 1970 and 13.3 in 1980. The *ages* at which terminations were carried out (Table 8) were mostly in the 20–34 year group.

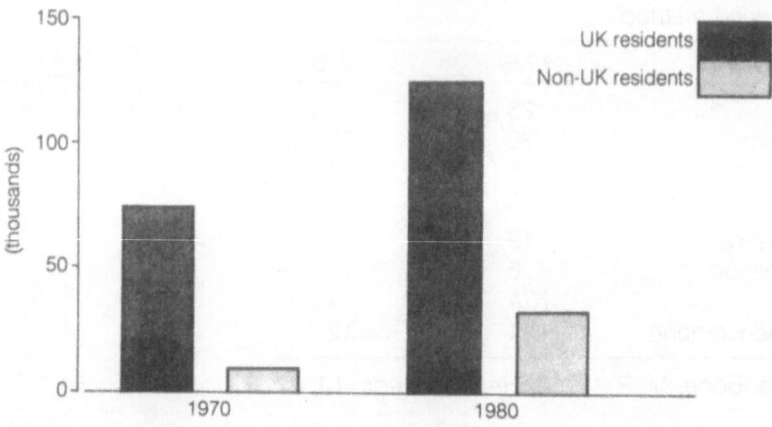

Figure 13   Termination of pregnancy, 1970 and 1980 (Health and Personal Social Services Statistics, *1982, Table 12.1)*

Table 7   Termination of pregnancy, 1970 and 1980

	1970		1980		Increase
	Numbers	*%*	*Numbers*	*%*	*1970–1980*
UK residents	72,127	87	126,642	79	×1.8
Non-UK residents	10,603	13	32,801	21	×3.0
Total	82,730	100	159,503	100	×1.9

Source: *Health and Personal Social Services Statistics*, 1982, Table 12.1

Table 8   Termination of pregnancy, 1980, by ages (England)

Age	Under 16	16–19	20–34	35–44	Others	Numbers
Percentage of all terminations	3	25	57	14	1	159,503

Source: *Health and Personal Social Services Statistics*, 1982, Table 12.1

Marital status

Table 9 shows that most women who had termination of pregnancy were single.

Table 9   Termination of pregnancy, by marital status and place of resident (England, 1980)

	Marital status		
Place of residence	Single	Married	Widowed/divorced/ separated and other
UK residents (%)	54	34	12
Non-UK residents (%)	64	30	6
All cases	58	32	10

Source: *Health and Personal Social Services Statistics*, 1982, Table 12.1

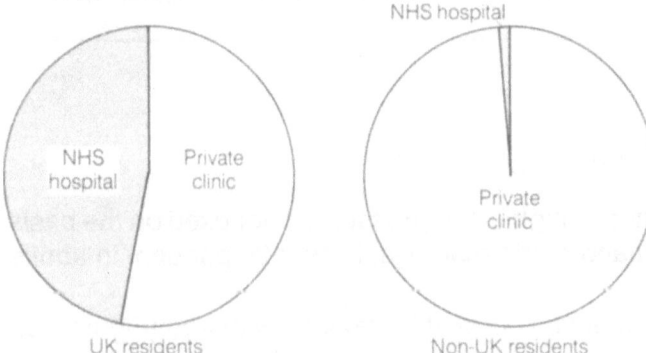

Figure 14   Termination of pregnancy, by place where carried out (England, 1980) (Health and Personal Social Services Statistics, 1982, Table 12.1)

Place where termination carried out
The private sector carries out the majority of terminations for UK residents, and almost all of non-UK residents (Figure 14 and Table 10).

Table 10   Termination of pregnancy, by place where carried out (England, 1980)

	NHS hospital	Private clinic or hospital
UK residents (%)	47	53
Non-UK residents (%)	1	99

Source: *Health and Personal Social Services Statistics*, 1982, Table 12.1

Self-check

In addition to large-scale epidemiological studies there is need for physicians, groups of physicians, hospitals and other units and districts to carry out occasional but regular audits or self-checks of outcomes of care. As examples, experiences over 30 years of recording and analysing data in a single British general practice (J.F.) summarize clinical outcomes in some selected conditions (Fry, J. *Common Diseases*, 3rd edition, 1983, Lancaster: MTP).

HIGH BLOOD PRESSURE

- The prevalence of high blood pressure, diagnosed on the basis of sphygmomanometric readings, is over 20 per cent in adults over 30.
- The age prevalence is one of increasing with age (Figure 15).
- One-half of all newly diagnosed hypertensives are over 60 years when first diagnosed.
- The SMRs are inversely related to age at diagnosis (Figure 16) (Fry, 1983, *op. cit.*).

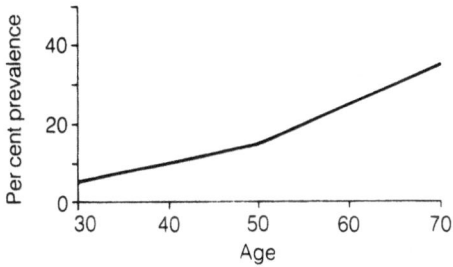

Figure 15   High blood pressure: age prevalence

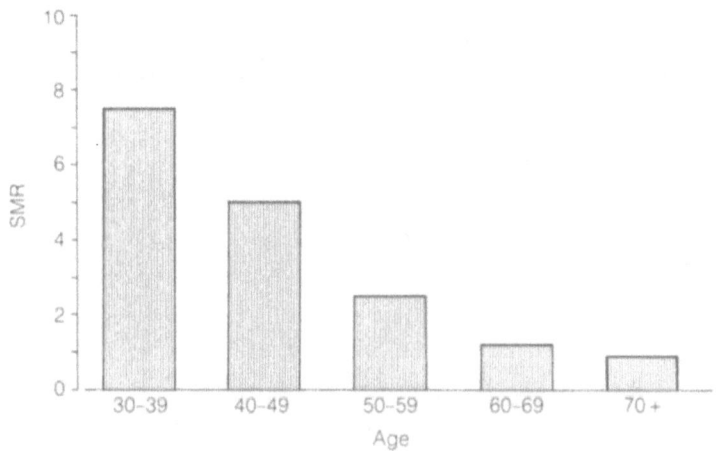

Figure 16   High blood pressure: SMRs related to age at diagnosis

- In hypertensives first diagnosed at 60 + , the expected mortality rates are scarcely above those expected.
- The major risk in hypertensives is death from stroke, and to a lesser extent from ischaemic heart disease (IHD) (Figure 17).
- A rule of 'one-halves' at present exists (Figure 18).
- One-half of all hypertensives in the community are undiagnosed.
- Of those diagnosed one-half are being treated.
- In those being treated, in one-half is the raised blood pressure controlled.

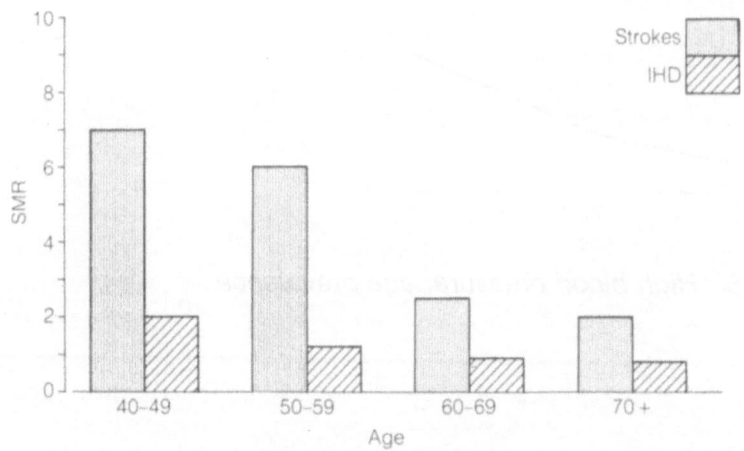

Figure 17   High blood pressure: SMRs for strokes and IHD

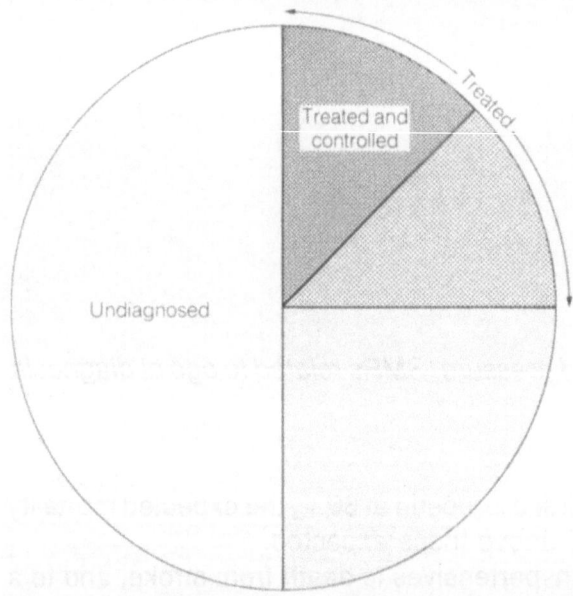

Figure 18   High blood pressure: 'rule of one-halves'

- The degrees of control (Figure 19) in those treated were 'good' (DBP below 90 mmHg) in 20 per cent, 'moderate' (DBP 90–110 mmHg) in 60 per cent and 'poor' in 20 per cent (DBP over 110 mmHg) (Figure 19) (Fry, 1981, *op. cit.*).

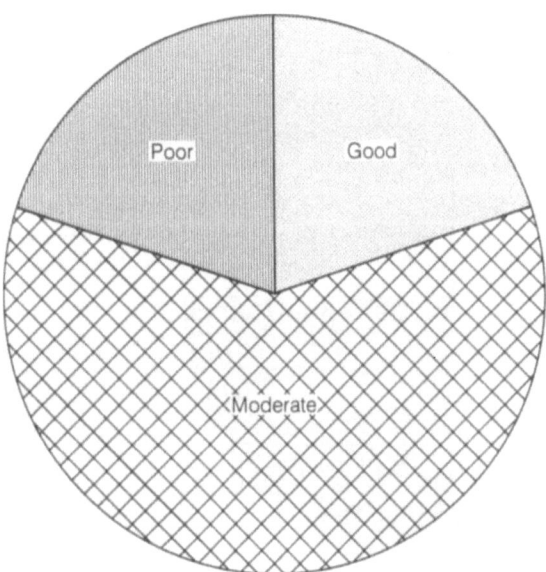

Figure 19   High blood pressure: degrees of control

- The issues raised are:
  - who should be treated for high blood pressure – if the SMRs in over-60s are no greater than expected?
  - how may control be made more effective?

DIABETES

- The prevalence of known diabetes is between 5 and 10 per 1000.
- Age prevalence goes up with age.
- The rule of one-halves also applies to diabetes (Figure 20):
  - one-half of all diabetics in a community have been diagnosed;
  - of known diabetics treated one-half are well controlled.

- The *degrees of control* (Figure 21):
  - 43 per cent *well controlled* (blood sugar below 10 mmol/l)
  - 39 per cent *moderate control* (blood sugar 10–19 mmol/l)
  - 18 per cent *poor control* (blood sugar above 20 mmol/l)

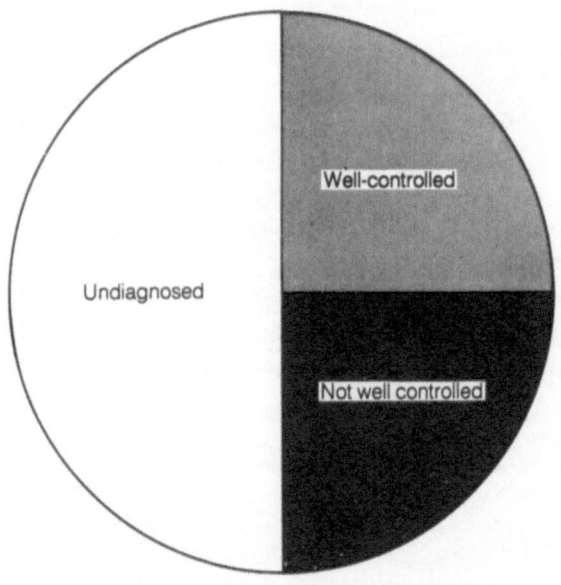

Figure 20   Diabetes: rule of one-halves

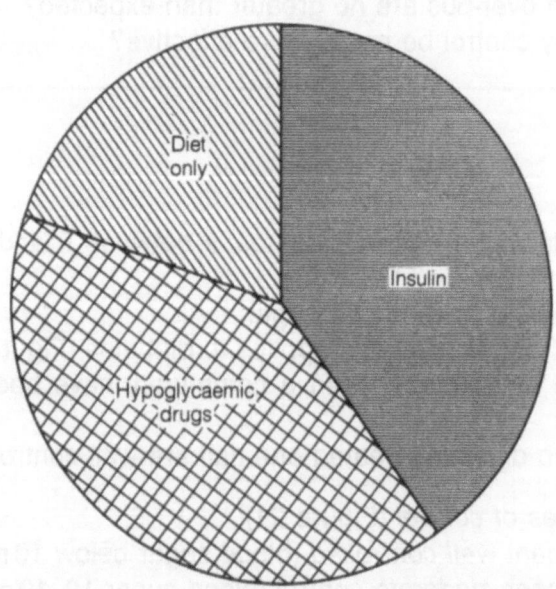

Figure 21   Diabetes: methods of management

- The *management of diabetes* (Figure 21):
  - diet only   20 per cent
  - hypoglycaemic drugs   40 per cent
  - insulin   40 per cent

THYROID DISORDERS

- Prevalence of known *hypothyroidism* is 5 per 1000, but as many may be undiagnosed in the community.
- Annual incidence of *hyperthyroidism* is 0.25 per 1000 per year.
- *Hypothyroidism* – well controlled (thyroid function tests) in 70 per cent.
- *Hyperthyroidism*:
  - post-treatment (surgery or radioactive iodine) *hypothyroidism* in 55 per cent.

PEPTIC ULCERS

- The annual prevalence (annual consulting rate) is 15 per 1000.
- For duodenal ulcers it is 12 per 1000 and for gastric ulcers 3 per 1000.
- Age prevalence for *duodenal ulcers* (Figure 22) suggests tendency to natural remission; that for *gastric ulcers* suggests continuing problems. One-half remit completely.

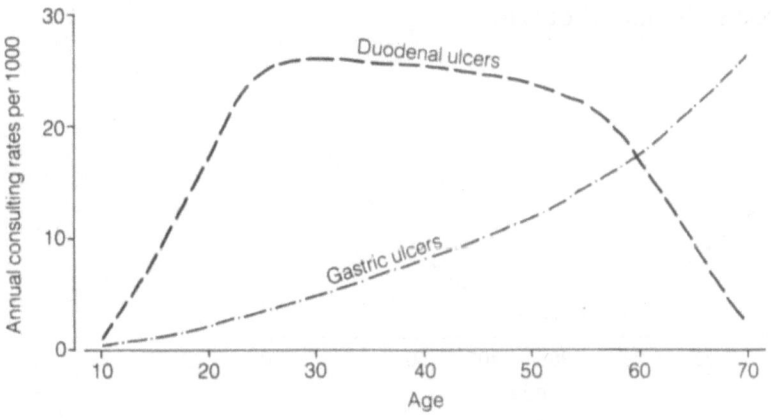

Figure 22   Peptic ulcers: age prevalence

- Outcomes on observation (over 30 years) (Figure 23) show tendency to natural improvement but with appreciable proportions needing surgery (probably less now with H₂ histamine antagonists).

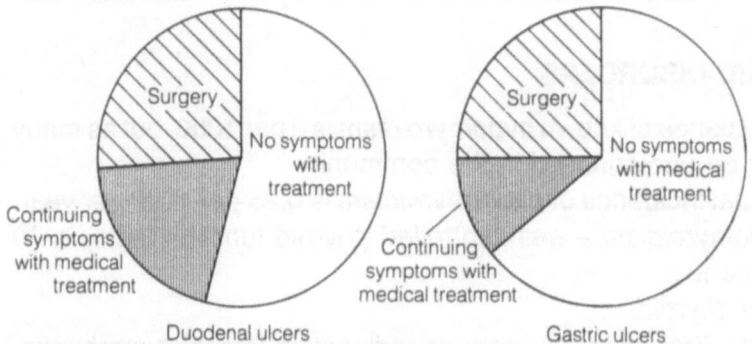

Figure 23   Peptic ulcers: outcomes

ACUTE WHEEZY CHESTS/ASTHMA

- *Acute wheezing chest* (AWC) is a physical sign and not a specific disease.
- Within it there are at least *three distinct clinical groups*:
  - AWC in 'catarrhal children';
  - AWC in chronic bronchitics;
  - asthma.
- *Age prevalence* for all acute wheezy chests/asthma (Figure 24) shows U-shaped curve.

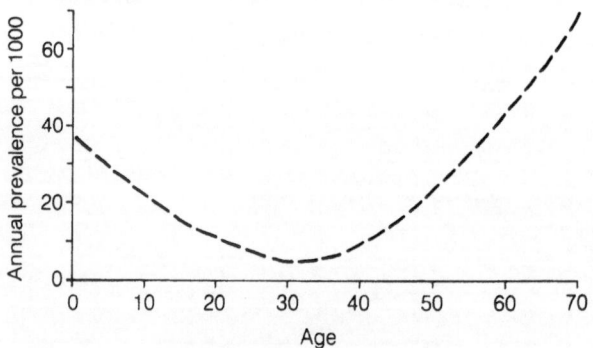

Figure 24   AWC/asthma: annual prevalence

- The annual age prevalence rates for the three clinical types are different (Figure 25).

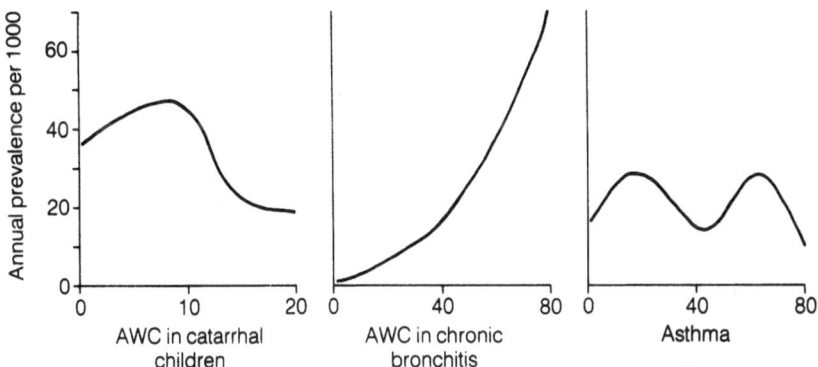

Figure 25   AWC/asthma: annual age prevalence

- *Outcomes* (Figure 26) show the differences in functional disabilities.

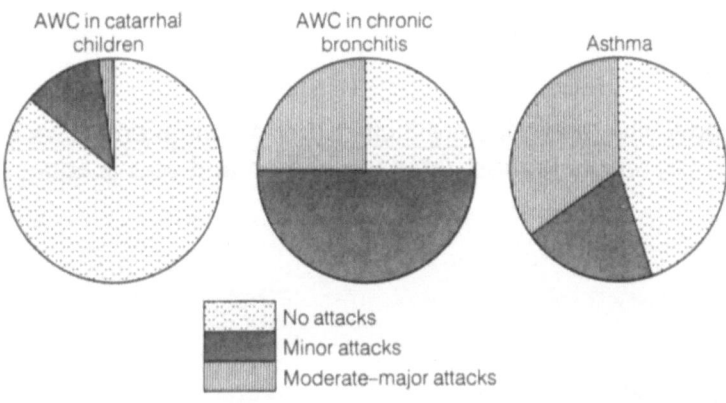

Figure 26   Acute wheezy chests/asthma – outcomes

RHEUMATOID ARTHRITIS

- Advances in medical and physical methods have not prevented considerable functional disability (Figure 27).

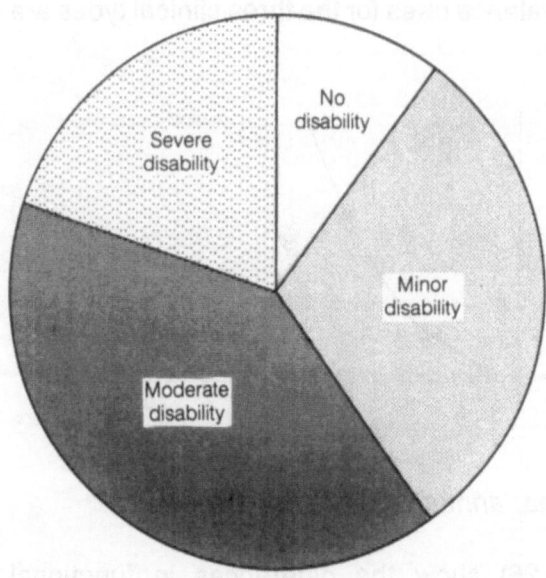

Figure 27   Rheumatoid arthritis: functional state at follow-up

EPILEPSY

- If all convulsive episodes are included, the *annual prevalence* (Figure 28) shows highest rates in children and young adults.

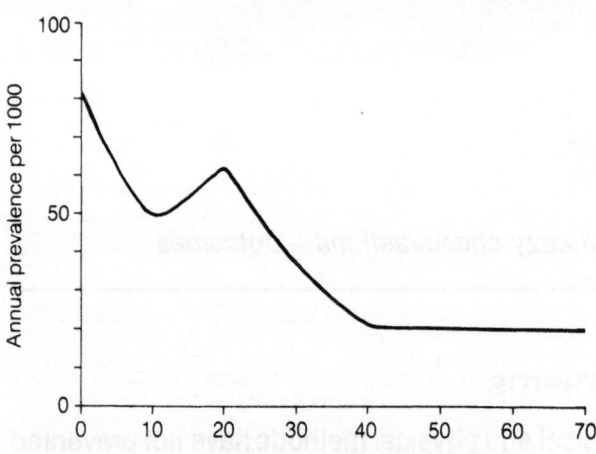

Figure 28   Epilepsy: annual prevalence

- The *outcomes* (Figure 29) show a good prognosis for convulsions occurring in first 15 years (including febrile convulsions) and a fair one for those commencing after the age of 15.

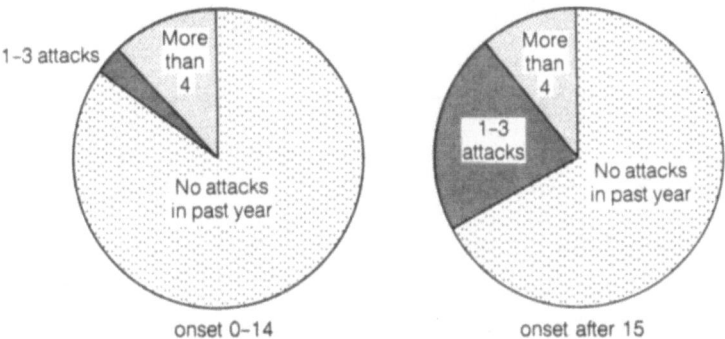

Figure 29 Epilepsy: outcomes – attacks in past year (follow-up 5 years +)

CANCERS

- Annual incidence of new cases: 3–4 per 1000.
- Although some cancers occur in younger persons, in general it tends to be associated with ageing (Figure 30).

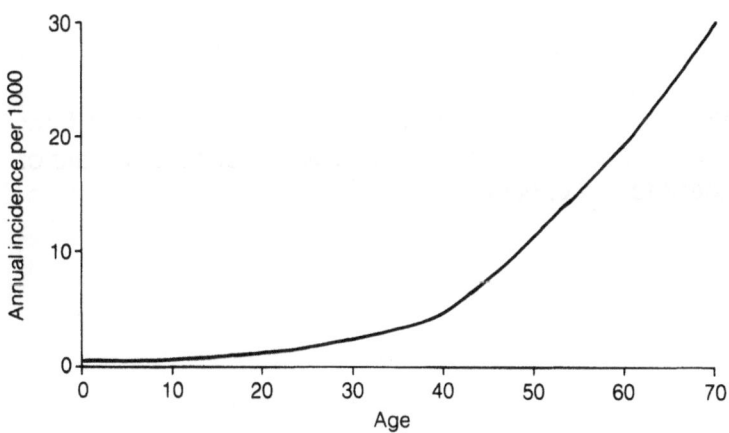

Figure 30 Cancers: annual age incidence

- The most prevalent types of cancers (Figure 31) are gastro-intestinal, bronchus–lung and breast.

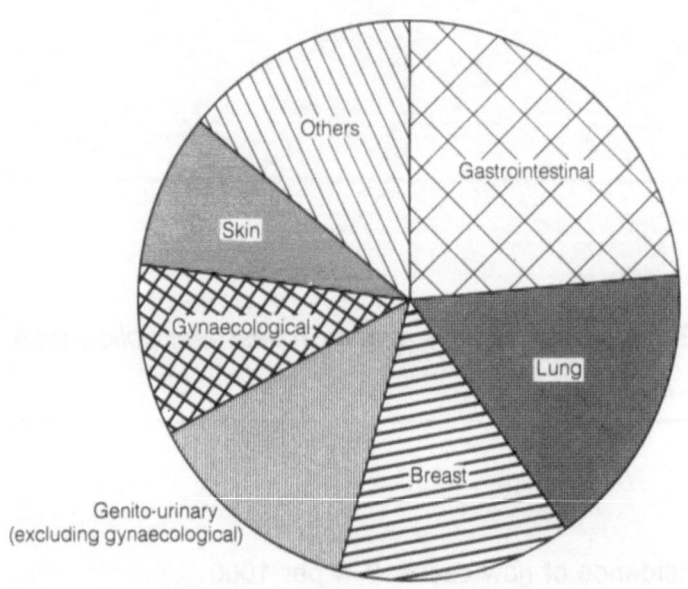

Figure 31   Cancers: proportions of frequency

- The 5-year survival rates (Figure 32 and Table 11) range from 100 per cent to almost nil with an *overall 5-year survival rate* of 36 per cent for all cancers.

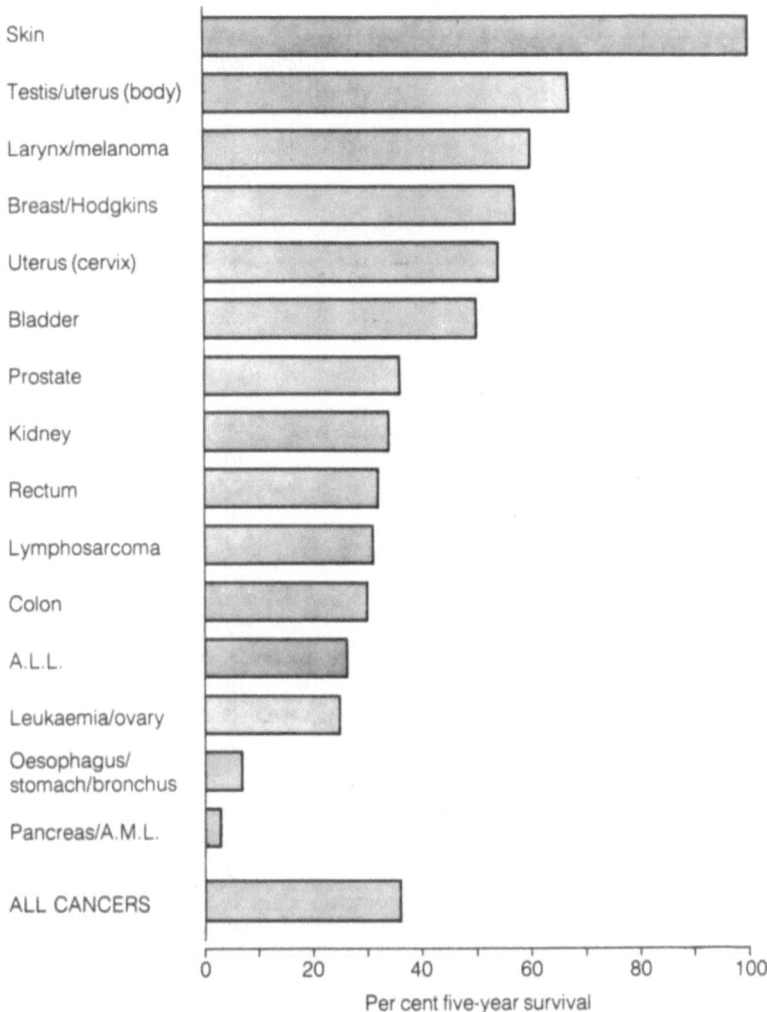

Figure 32   Cancers: 5-year survivals

Table 11   Cancers: 5-year survivals

Site	5-year survival (percentage of cases)
Skin (excluding melanoma)	100
Testis	67
Uterus (corpus)	67
Larynx	60
Melanoma	60
Breast	57
Hodgkins	57
Cervix uterus	54
Bladder	50
Prostate	36
Kidney	34
Rectum	32
Lymphosarcoma	31
Colon	30
Acute lymphatic leukaemia (A.L.L.)	27
Non-acute leukaemias	25
Ovary	25
Oesophagus	7
Stomach	7
Bronchus–lung	7
Pancreas	3
Acute myeloid leukaemia (A.M.L.)	3
All cancers	36

Source:

COMMENT

- *Cervical cytology* is increasing, but in 1980 the smears examined accounted for 25 per cent of women in the 15–50 age group. There is no information on percentage having an examination every 5 years.

- Abnormal smears are found in 7 per 1000 smears examined.
- A decline in registration of, and mortality from, cervical cancer has occurred.
- Acceptance rates for *immunization* of children are insufficient for control of the infection:
  - for diphtheria, tetanus and polio it is around 80 per cent;
  - for whooping cough it is 45 per cent;
  - for measles it is 55 per cent;
  - for rubella it is 84 per cent.
- Thirty-seven per cent of women age 15–44 received *family planning advice* from GPs and community family planning clinics;
- More than one-half received it from GPs.
- Eighty per cent of women use family planning in the early period of marriage.
- The 'pill' is the most popular form of contraception.
- *Termination* of *pregnancy*: numbers doubled, 1970–1980.
- Of all terminations 57 per cent are for women aged 20–34 and 25 per cent for the 16–19 age group.
- Of those undergoing termination 32 per cent are married, 58 per cent single and 10 per cent in 'other' category.
- Of UK residents 47 per cent of terminations are in NHS hospitals and 53 per cent in private clinics.
- A process of *'self-check'* illustrates some questionable results:
  - *hypertension* is not well controlled;
  - *diabetes* is not well controlled;
  - *thyrotoxicosis*: one-half become hypothyroid after treatment;
  - *peptic ulcers*: more than one-half are 'cured' with simple medical measures;
  - *cancers*: 5-year survival rate for all cancers is 36 per cent;
  - *rheumatoid arthritis*: results are poor;
  - *epilepsy*: outcome good;
  - *asthma*: outcome good.
- The importance of measurement and evaluation of *quality of care* is inestimable; it has received insufficient attention in the NHS.

Self-check of a Specialty: Anaesthetic Deaths

IAN McCOLL

The best known continuing assessment of clinical quality of care are the confidential enquiries carried out by the Department of Health and Social Security.

The Association of Anaesthetists reported on *Mortality Associated with Anaesthesia* (J. N. Lunn and W. W. Mushin, 1982, London: Nuffield Provincial Hospitals Trust).

This was not a comprehensive national survey but restricted to five regions with 6060 deaths within six days of over 1 million surgical operations. The retrieval rate was 62 per cent. Therefore the findings must be pointers and not complete pictures based on 3736 operations.

The six-day post-operative death rate was 5.3 per 1000 operations. 10 per cent of these were attributed in whole or in part to anaesthesia, a rate of 0.53 per 1000 operations, one in 1900 surgical operations (Figure 33). The rates are very low but one-third are avoidable (page 229).

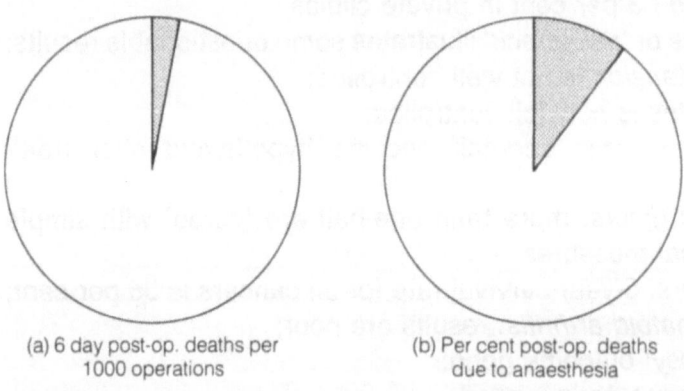

(a) 6 day post-op. deaths per
1000 operations

(b) Per cent post-op. deaths
due to anaesthesia

Figure 33   6-day post-operative deaths (a) per 1000 surgical operations (b) percentage of all post-operative deaths due to anaesthesia

THE PATIENT

Age

The majority of post-operative anaesthetic deaths were elderly –
one-half over 70 and three-quarters over 60, but 3 per cent were
under 10 years of age (Figure 34).

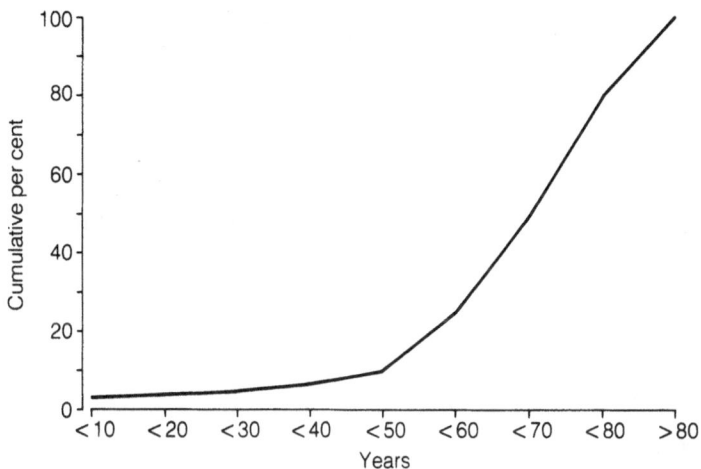

Figure 34   Age at death: cumulative percentage

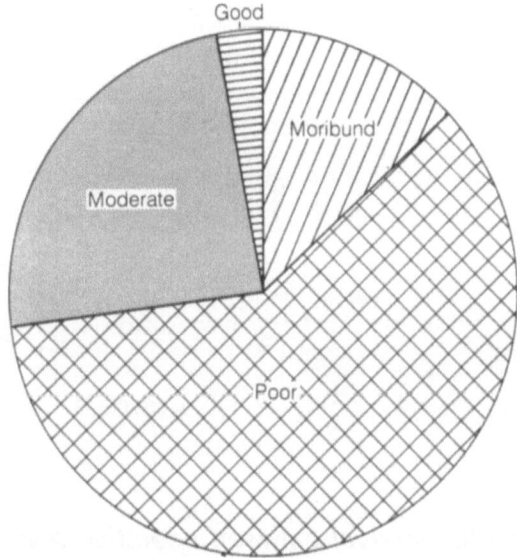

Figure 35   Anaesthetic deaths: pre-operative state

Preoperative state of the patient

Nearly three-quarters of the anaesthetic deaths were in those assessed as in poor or moribund conditions and only 3 per cent were in a good pre-operative state (Figure 35).

Type of surgery performed

One-half of cases were 'elective' and one-half were 'emergencies'.

Time of death

More than one-third (38 per cent) died on the same day as the operation and by end of day one, two-thirds had died (Figure 36).

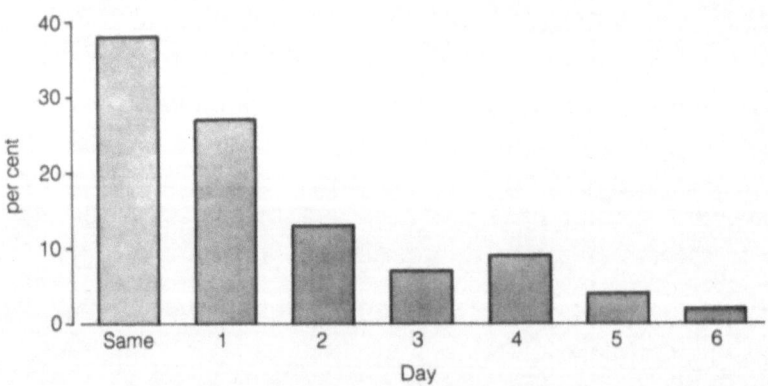

Figure 36   Anaesthetic deaths: interval between operation and death

Place of death

More than one-half (52 per cent) died in the ward which is surprising. One-quarter (25 per cent) died in an intensive therapy unit and 16 per cent in the theatre and 5 per cent in a recovery room (Figure 37).

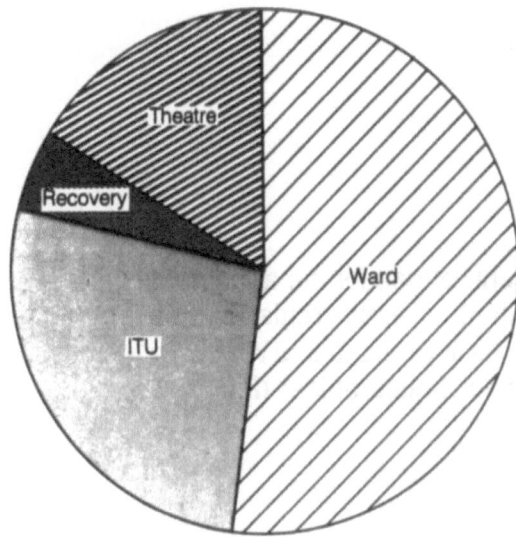

Figure 37   Anaesthetic deaths: location at death

Cause of death

The autopsy rate was only 42 per cent, a low rate on which to make judgments.
Of those autopsied, causes of death were reported as

	%
Cardio-vascular	45
Pulmonary	28 (pulmonary emboli 8)
Cerebral	9
Neoplastic disease	8
Miscellaneous	10
	100

THE ANAESTHETIST

Age

40 per cent were under 35
50 per cent were 35–54
10 per cent were over 55

Grade

In over one-half (62 per cent) of deaths the anaesthetic had been administered by a consultant or senior registrar; this is a higher proportion than anaesthetists in England and Wales. In 14 per cent, the anaesthetist was a senior house officer (Figure 38).

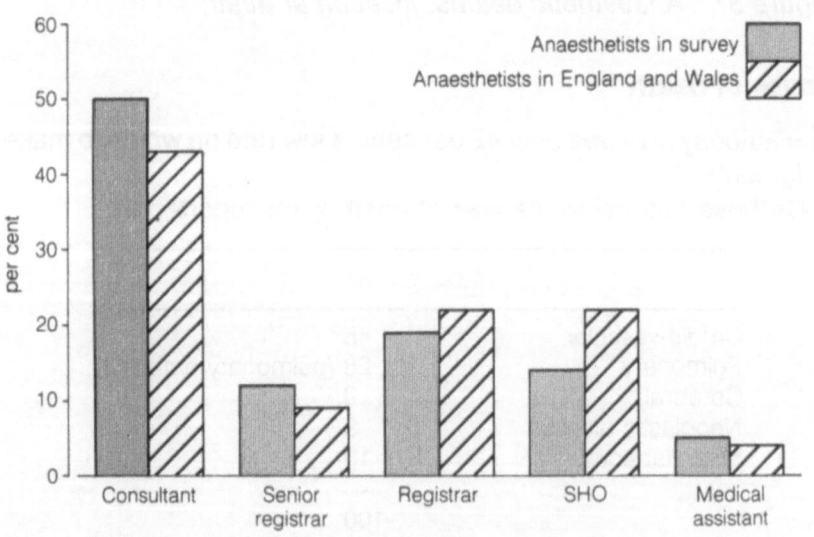

Figure 38 Anaesthetic deaths: grade of anaesthetist

Experience

45 per cent had more than 10 years anaesthetic experience
23 per cent had 5–9 years anaesthetic experience
16 per cent had 2–4 years anaesthetic experience
16 per cent had less than 2 years anaesthetic experience
Note that one-third of those anaesthetizing in cases of anaesthetic deaths had less than 5 years experience.

Anaesthetic management

Of certain specialized anaesthetic procedures analysed, it is reported that:
- assistance for the anaesthetist was available from other anaesthetists, nurses and technicians
- instrumental monitoring was inadequate
- clinical anaesthetic records were not always kept
- there were no recovery rooms in 18 per cent of cases.

ASSESSORS' OPINIONS

Contribution of anaesthesia to death

Anaesthesia was totally responsible in 16 per cent of deaths and partly responsible in 46 per cent (Figure 39).

Deficiencies

The assessors concluded that:
- clinical failure occurred in 43 per cent
- organizational failure occurred in 35 per cent.

Avoidability of death

It was considered that 34 per cent of anaesthetic deaths were avoidable (Figure 40).

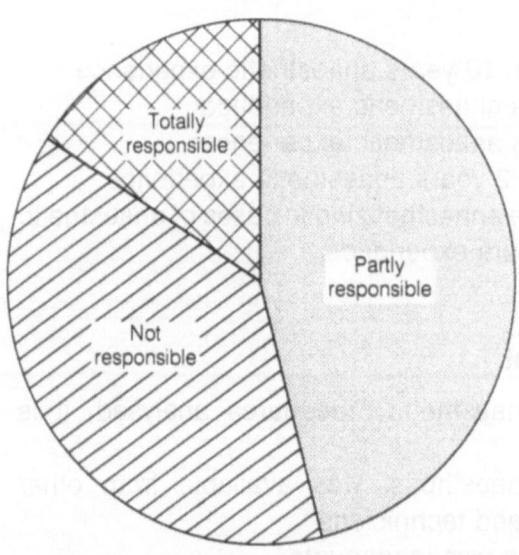

Figure 39   Anaesthetic deaths: extent of anaesthetic involvement

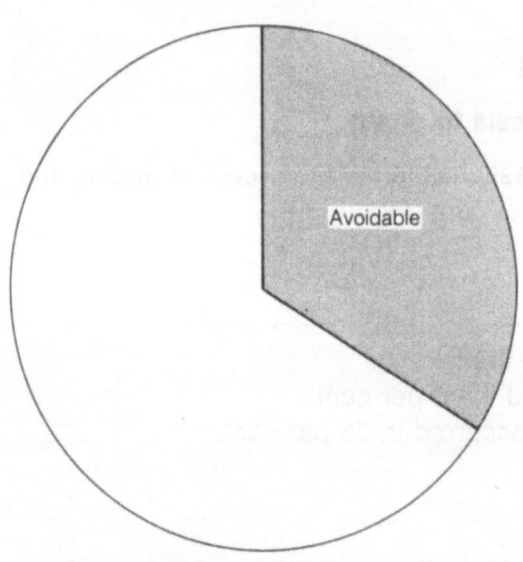

Figure 40   Anaesthetic deaths: avoidability

Avoidable factors in anaesthetic deaths were assessed as:

	%
Lack of experience	30
Lack of assistance	10
Error of judgment	70
Error of clinical expertise	36
Error of technical expertise	24
Lack of equipment	7
Failure of equipment	5

COMMENT

The authors' summary in the report includes conclusions:
- the process of anaesthesia is remarkably safe.
- nevertheless there are probably almost 300 avoidable anaesthetic deaths in Britain annually.
- mistakes occur in all grades of anaesthetists but trainees are too often left unsupported by consultants.
- essential monitoring equipment is inadequate.
- clinical anaesthetic records are not always kept.
- in some hospitals recovery facilities are not available.
- there is little evidence that fatigue of the anaesthetist plays much part in the deaths.
- there appears to be insufficient consultation between anaesthetist and surgeon.

Continuing Check on the Outcome of Dialysis and Transplantation

IAN McCOLL

Renal specialists are considered to have done more than any other group of clinicians to monitor their performance. Through a European Registry, they have now collected a comprehensive array of data on the outcome of dialysis and transplantation in 35

European countries, including the UK. Annual reviews appear in the *Proceedings of the European Dialysis and Transplant Association* (edited by B. H. B. Robinson, 1982, London: Pitman Books Limited) and in the *U.K. Transplant Service Review* (edited by B. Bradley and D. Moras, 1982, Bristol: UK Transplant Service).

Stock of patients

By the end of 1981 a stock of more than 8,000 UK patients were being kept alive on treatment for end stage renal failure. This is equivalent to 143.2 per million population (pmp) compared with 127.8 pmp in 1980 and 31.8 pmp in 1971 (Figure 41).

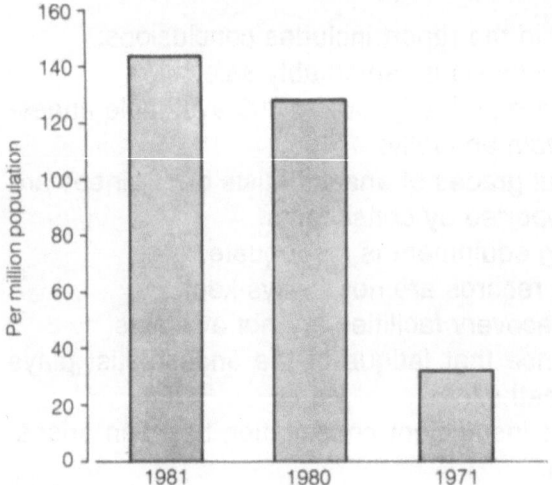

Figure 41 Patients alive on renal replacement therapy at December 1981

Patient flow

The flow of patients during 1981 is shown in Figure 42.
- 1,422 new patients (25.4 pmp) were accepted for treatment
- 531 deaths (9.5 pmp) occurred, offsetting intake by nearly one-third
- 877 transplants were performed, a rate of 15.7 pmp.

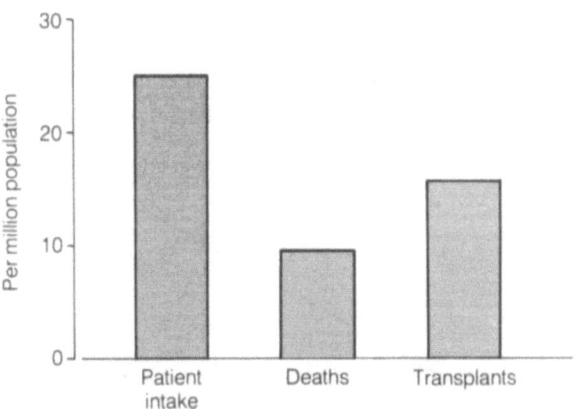

Figure 42   Patient flow during 1981

Patient intake vs need

At 25.4 per million population, patient intake falls short of the most conservative estimate of need (40 pmp per year) and it falls far below the all inclusive estimate of need (150 pmp per year) shown in Figure 43.

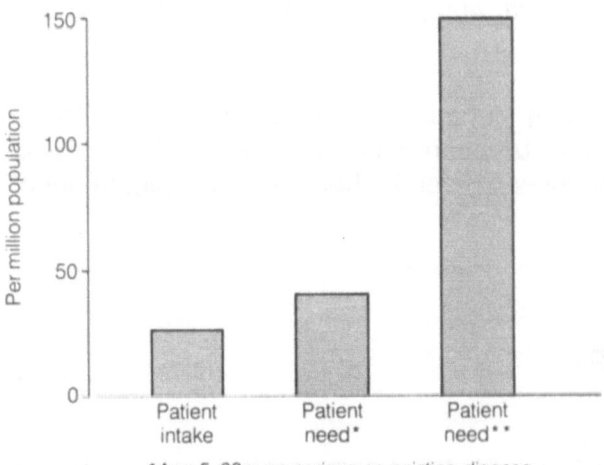

*Age 5–60 y, no serious co-existing disease
**All ages and all conditions

Figure 43   Patient intake vs need

Transplantation vs need

There is also a considerable shortfall between transplantation activity (transplants actually carried out) and the number of patients awaiting transplants (Figure 44).

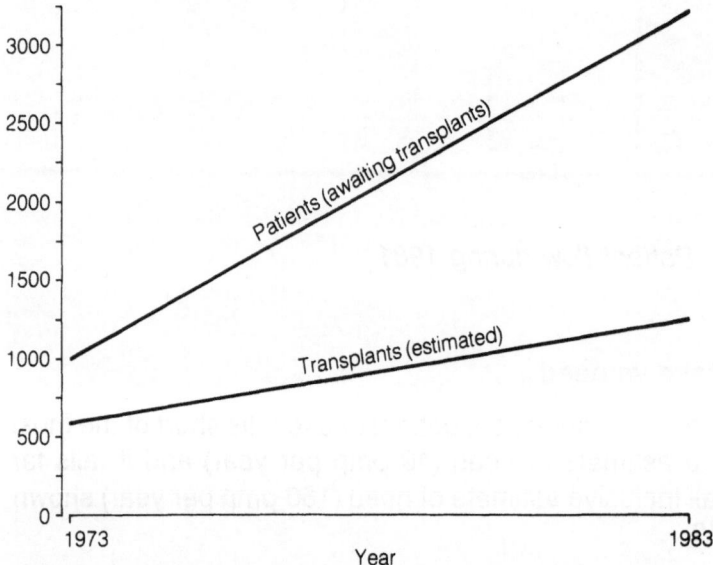

Figure 44   Transplant rate and patient need between 1973 and 1983 in UK

Note: Ranked according to patient intake each year, the UK is seventeenth out of 35 European countries, but ranked by transplantation rate it occupies a much higher position, seventh out of 25 countries.

MODE OF THERAPY

Transplants

More patients owe their lives to functioning grafts than to any other single form of renal replacement therapy, 53 per cent being kept alive on grafts compared with 42 per cent on all forms of dialysis (Figure 45).

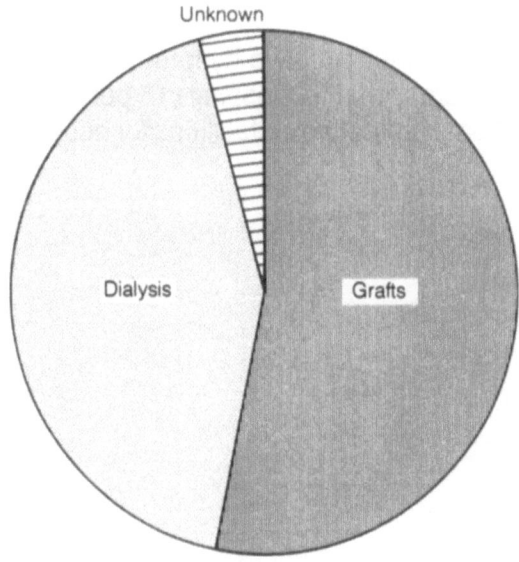

Figure 45   Patients alive on grafts and on dialysis (1981)

Type of graft

Most of the grafts (81 per cent) come from cadavers, 12 per cent are from living donors. Retransplantation accounts for 14 per cent of all grafts (Figure 46).

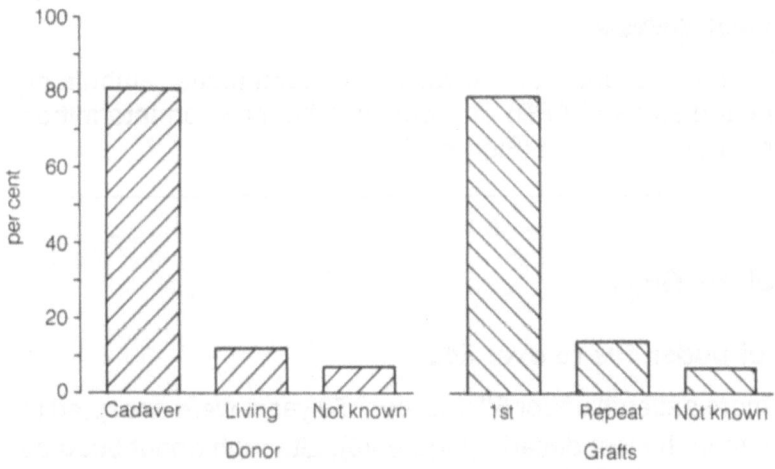

Figure 46   Cadaver vs living donors and 1st vs repeat grafts (1981)

Haemodialysis

In 42 per cent of cases, patients are kept alive by haemodialysis, mainly at home (26 per cent) rather than in hospital (16 per cent), reflecting the continuing national restriction on facilities for hospital haemodialysis (Figure 47).

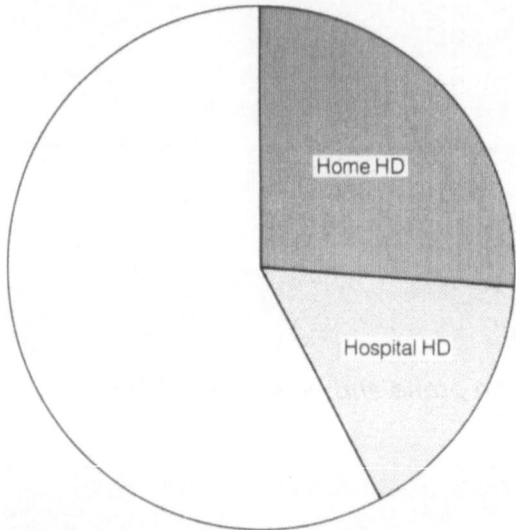

Figure 47   % of patients alive on home and on hospital haemodialysis (1981)

Peritoneal dialysis

One in ten patients are treated by continuous ambulatory peritoneal dialysis (CAPD) and one in a hundred on intermittent peritoneal dialysis (IPD) (Figure 48).

AGE OF PATIENT

Ratio of under 50s to over 50s

Many more patients under 50 than over 50 years were accepted for treatment in the last decade (Figure 49), although about 6000 out of the estimated 7500 patients who suffer renal failure each year are over 55 years, as renal failure increases sharply with age.

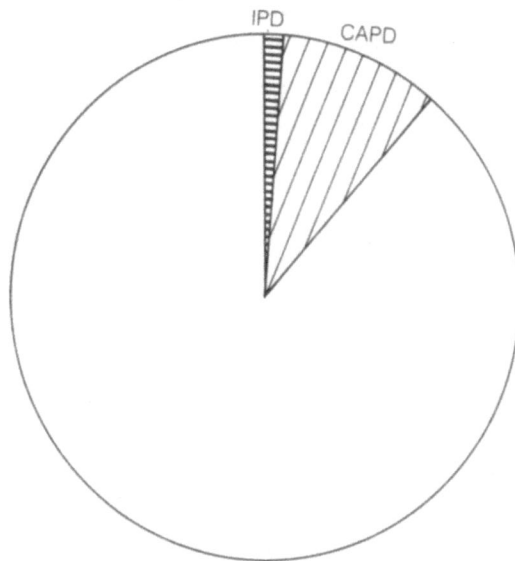

Figure 48   % of patients alive on CAPD and on IPD (1981)

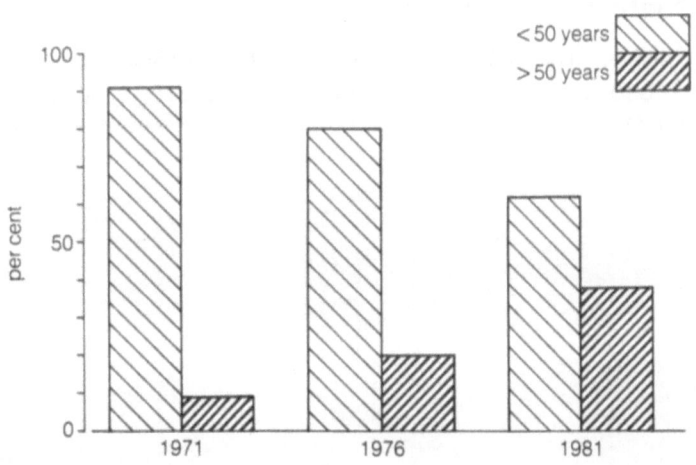

Figure 49   Ratio of patients under 50 to over 50 years

Average age

The average age of patients accepted for treatment rose from 35 years in 1971 to 42 years in 1981 (Figure 50), but it still compares unfavourably with many other European countries.

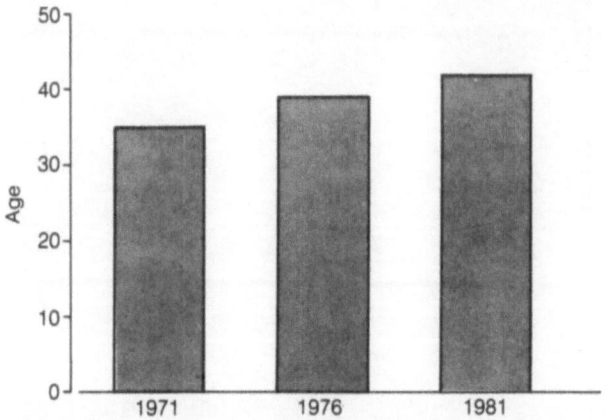

Figure 50   Average age of patients accepted for therapy

Average age and mode of therapy

Patients on functioning grafts show the lowest average age, 39 years, while those on CAPD record the highest average age, 48 years (Figure 51).

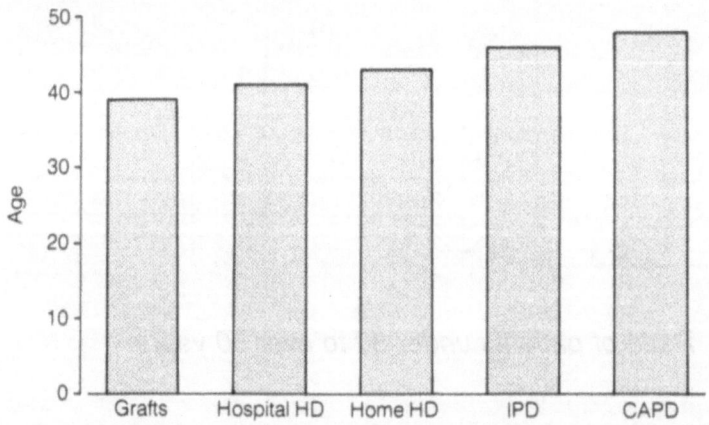

Figure 51   Average age of patient and mode of therapy (1981)

238   QUALITY AND OUTCOMES

PATIENT SURVIVAL AT FIVE YEARS

Improved survival

Patients who commenced treatment in the second half of the 1970s show noticeably better survival at five years compared with those who began treatment in the early 1970s (Figure 52). This is despite the older average age of more recent patients which might be expected to have resulted in poorer survival prospects.

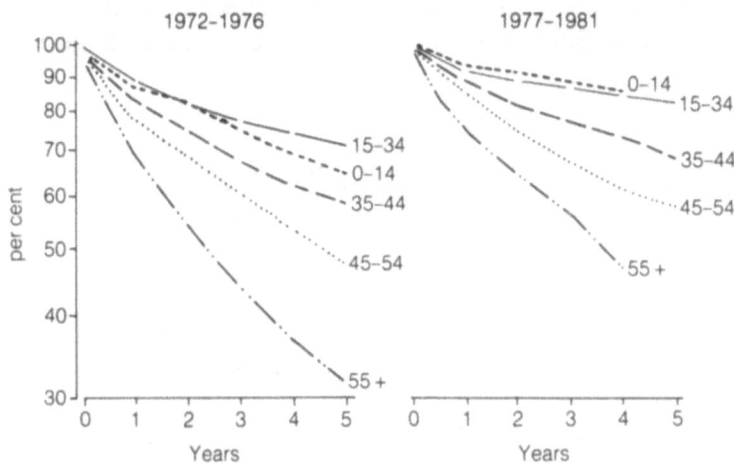

Figure 52   Improved 5-year survival on all modes of therapy combined (actuarial calculation, per cent plus standard error)

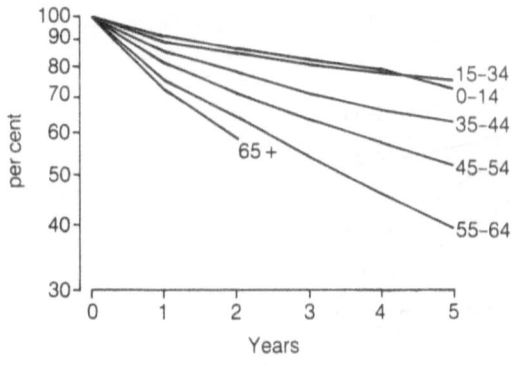

Figure 53   Age and 5-year cumulative survival on all forms of therapy: 1974 onwards

Age and survival

However, the age at which patients begin treatment is still an important influence on outcome. After 35 years, survival decreases with increasing age (Figure 53), reflecting increased susceptibility both to natural death and to therapeutic complications.

Transplantation vs dialysis

Patients who received grafts show slightly higher survival rates at five years (Figure 54a), even if they needed to be changed to

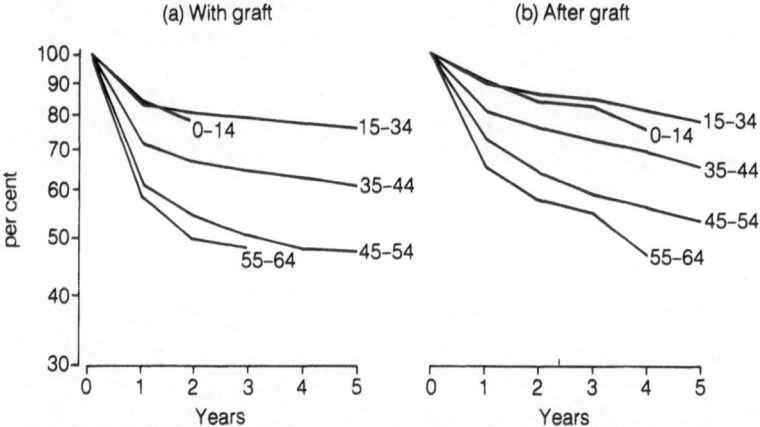

Figure 54   5-year cumulative survival (a) with 1st cadaver graft and (b) after graft

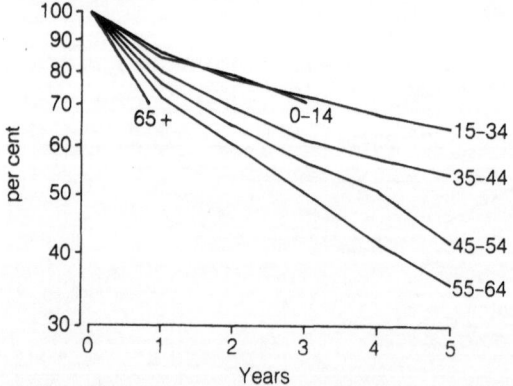

Figure 55   5-year cumulative survival on home and hospital haemodialysis: 1974 onwards

dialysis or received second and third grafts (Figure 54b), compared with patients whose sole mode of therapy was haemodialysis at home or in hospital (Figure 55).

PATIENT SURVIVAL AT ONE, TWO AND THREE YEARS

Four therapies compared

There are four main points to note in Figure 56:
- the results at one year reflect the higher mortality risk associated with transplantation in the early postoperative period, especially in patients receiving cadaver grafts, compared with the group on home haemodialysis
- the superior outcome on living donor grafts compared with cadaver grafts demonstrates the undoubted advantage of receiving a kidney from a relative
- moreover, once the difficult first year was passed, living donor grafts gave the best result of all therapies
- the higher survival rates for home haemodialysis compared with hospital haemodialysis is generally thought to reflect the selection of fitter patients for home therapy.

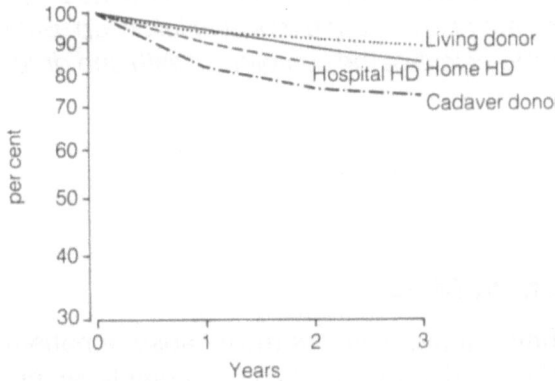

Figure 56 Four modes of therapy compared for short-term cumulative survival: 1977–1979

CAPD

There has been a dramatic increase in the use of CAPD since its introduction in the late 1970s (Figure 57a). But there has also been a high drop out rate, only 29 per cent of patients remaining on this therapy at two years, and reflecting a cumulative death rate of 25 per cent and a cumulative drop out rate of 61 per cent (Figure 57b).

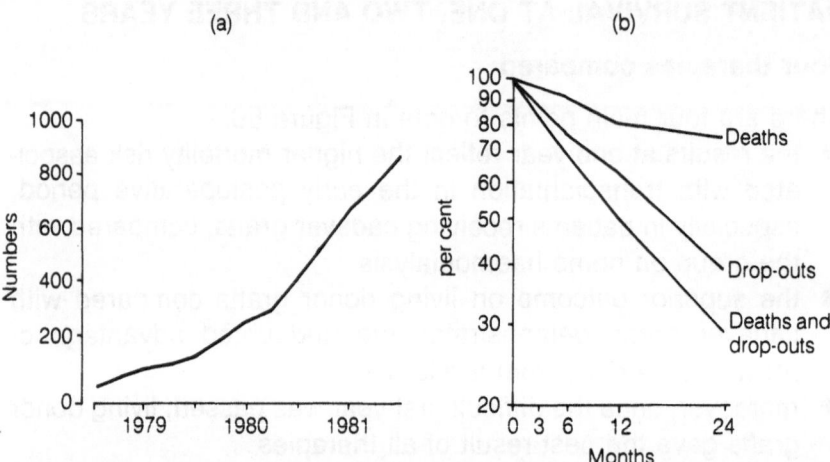

Figure 57 (a) Increase in use of CAPD and (b) two year survival

Note: In the death rate calculation in Figure 57b, patients who dropped-out are excluded as being lost to follow-up, and in the drop-out rate patients who died are also excluded as lost to follow-up. Both types of patients are used to calculate the combined death and drop-out rate.

Reasons for drop out from CAPD

Apart from transfer to other treatments, the main cause of patient drop out was peritonitis and other abdominal complications, accounting for 40 per cent of abandonments in the first year and 31 per cent in the second year (Figure 58).

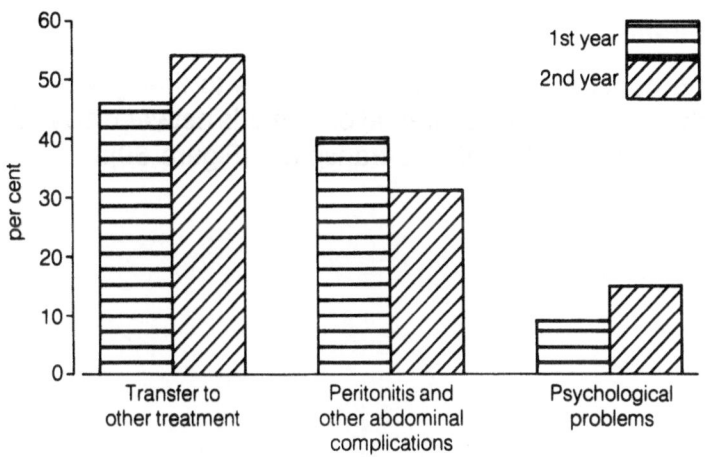

Figure 58   Reasons for abandoning CAPD

GRAFT SURVIVAL

Improved graft survival

Graft survival has also continued to improve with time, being 68 per cent at one year in 1981 compared with 49 per cent in 1972. But, as might be expected, it is still lower than patient survival, there being almost a 20 per cent difference in 1981 (Figure 59).

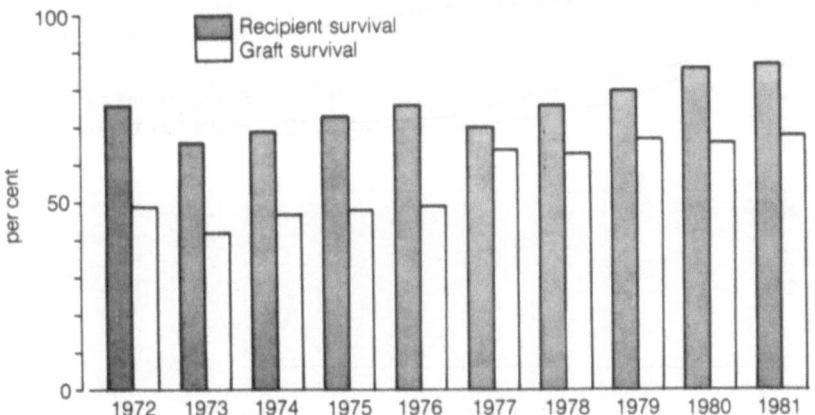

Figure 59   Graft cumulative survival at one year vs. patient survival: 1972–1981

Re-transplantation

Repeat grafts generally give far inferior results to first grafts. In most years the survival of a first graft at one year is between 10 and 20 per cent better than that of a re-transplant (Figure 60).

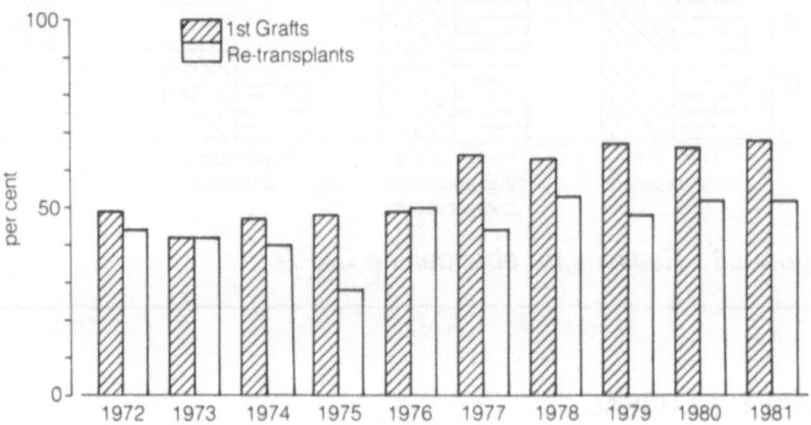

Figure 60   1st graft vs. repeat graft: cumulative survival at one year: 1972–1981

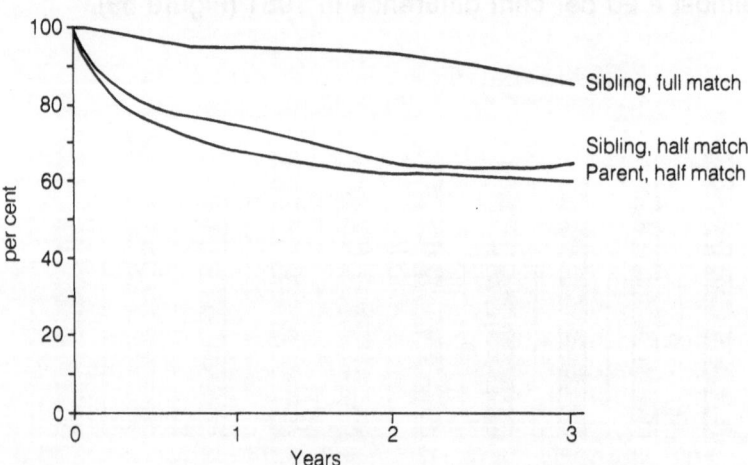

Figure 61   Full matched sibling grafts compared with half matched grafts from siblings or parents

244   QUALITY AND OUTCOMES

Living donor grafts

The outcome of tissue typing to reduce graft rejection has been very successful for living related donor grafts. Survival at one year ranges from 80 to 100 per cent for HLA identical grafts, when the two possible haplotypes are matched for donor and recipient, and from 80 to 62 per cent for partially matched living donor grafts, when only one of the two possible haplotypes are matched (Figure 61).

Living donor vs. cadaver grafts

But even when living donor grafts can be only partially matched, survival is still usually higher than that for cadaver grafts (Figure 62).

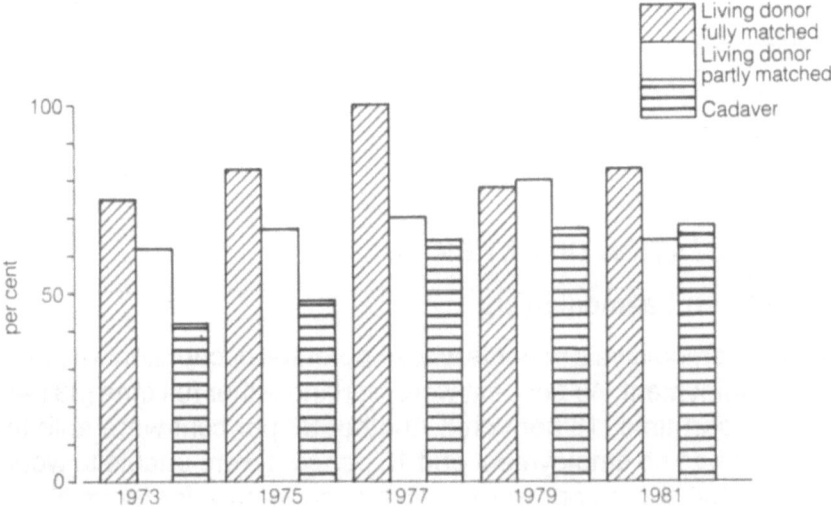

Figure 62 Cadaver vs. identical and partially matched living donor grafts: cumulative survival at one year

Type of graft and age of recipient

The highly successful outcome for living donor grafts is also thought to reflect in part the younger age of their recipients, who tend to be under 35 years, compared with the recipients of cadaver grafts, who tend to be over 35 years (Figure 63).

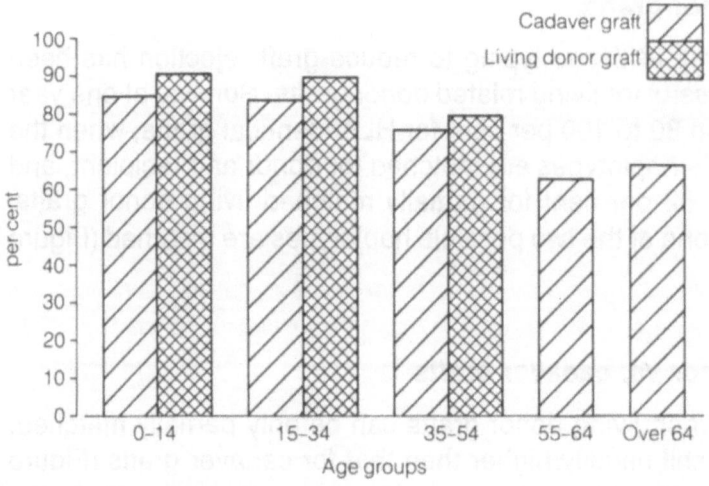

Figure 63   Age of recipient and type of graft: cumulative survival at one year

---

REHABILITATION OF PATIENTS

Patients on haemodialysis

Of the haemodialysis patients whose potential occupation was full-time employment, 49 per cent were working either full time (33 per cent) or part time (16 per cent). Another 33 per cent were able to work but had no employment and 15 per cent were unable to work and another 3 per cent were unable even to care for themselves (Figure 64).

Patients on functioning grafts

Of the patients on functioning grafts whose potential occupation was full-time employment, 81 per cent were working full time and 3 per cent part time. Another 11 per cent were able to work but were not in employment. Only four per cent were unable to work (Figure 64).

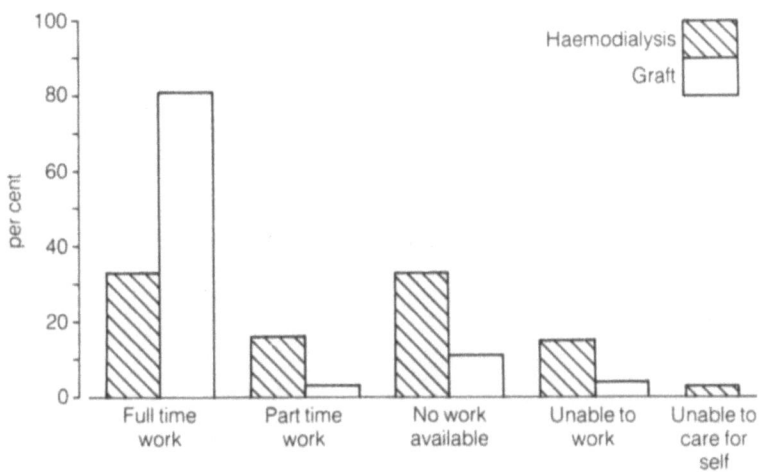

Figure 64   Rehabilitation of patients on haemodialysis and in grafts in 1979

CHAPTER 17

COMPLAINTS

The complaints procedures against registered medical practitioners are extensive. There are available to the public many channels of *complaint*:

- the Courts for civil actions;
- General Medical Council (GMC);
- Family Practitioner Committee (FPC);
- District Health Authorities (DHAs);
- Ombudsman;
- the public media;
- others, such as members of parliament and non-statutory and voluntary organizations.

It is difficult to know the extent of *dissatisfaction* amongst the public against the health services since such subjective feelings are difficult to measure.

Table 1 Annual numbers of complaints against doctors (estimated)

Body to whom complaint is made	Annual complaints
GMC	1000*
FPC	720†
DHA and others	6603‡
Total	8323
RMPs at risk	70,000
Percentage of all doctors	12%

Annual Report of GMC, for 1983.
†Health and Social Services Statistics, 1982, Table 5.14).
‡*Hansard*, 1 March 1983 (quoted in *British Medical Journal*, 1983, 1, 986)

There are over 70,000 registered medical practitioners (RMP) in clinical practice, and there are an estimated number of up to 8300 complaints against them annually (Table 1). The majority of the complaints noted in the table remain unproven but, nevertheless, they represent a level of dissatisfaction.

In an annual complaint rate against RMPs of 12 per cent, it is likely that each RMP may have more than one complaint in his/her professional lifetime.

General Medical Council (GMC)

The GMC is a statutory body set up in 1858 to promote and maintain standards in the medical profession. One of its roles is to receive complaints against RMPs and to decide if there is evidence of 'serious professional misconduct'. The disciplinary process of the GMC is one of stages:

1. *Complaint received.*
2. Complaint processed by *GMC staff.*
3. Referral to *preliminary screener*, whose function is to decide whether the complaint goes further.
4. Referral to *Preliminary Proceedings Committee*, which decides whether the case can be dealt with there by a letter of advice, or whether it should be referred to the Professional Conduct Committee.
5. *Professional Conduct Committee* meets in public and hears defence and prosecution against an RMP accused of possible serious professional misconduct.

The annual reports of the GMC give the size, nature and outcome of the complaints made. Table 2 and Figure 1 show the numbers

Table 2   GMC: annual numbers of complaints received, and their progress

	Numbers	Percentage
Complaints received	1000	100
Referred to Preliminary Proceedings Committee	120	12
Referred to Professional Conduct Committee	26	2.6

Source: From *Annual Reports of GMC*, 1973–1983

at each stage. They show also that less than 3 per cent of the complaints end in a public disciplinary hearing. From Table 2 and Figure 1 it is estimated that a RMP has only a 1 in 3000 chance of ever appearing before the Professional Conduct Committee of the GMC.

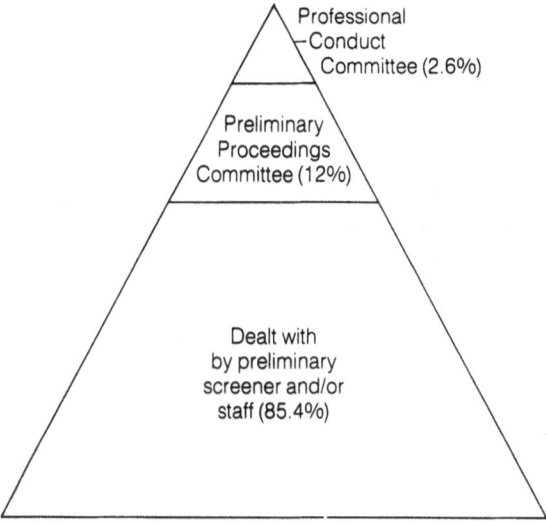

Figure 1   GMC: annual number of complaints received, and their progress

The *nature of the complaints against RMPs dealt with by the GMC* are shown in Tables 3 and 4, and Figure 2. Table 3 relates to the work of the *Preliminary Proceedings Committee*. The most frequent complaints are, in order:

- abuse of alcohol (most often conviction of drunken driving);
- dishonesty and improper financial dealings;
- personal abuse of drugs.

Note that disregard of personal patient care accounts for only 5 per cent of complaints.

Table 3   GMC: Preliminary Proceedings Committee: types of case

Complaint	Percentage
Disregard of personal patient care	5
Personal abuse of alcohol	27
Personal abuse of drugs	13
Improper prescribing of drugs	4
Breach of confidentiality	1
Improper sexual or emotional relations with patients	4
Dishonesty, etc.	18
Violence	4
Indecency	5
Advertising/canvassing	5
False certification	3
Others	11

Source: *Annual Reports of GMC*, 1973–1983

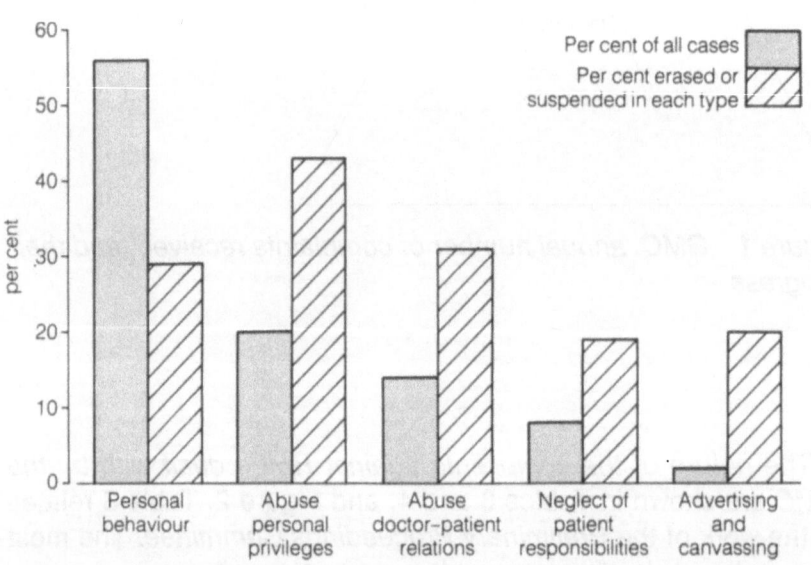

Figure 2   GMC: Professional Conduct Committee (Annual Reports of GMC, *1973–1983*)

The proportions of cases heard by the *Professional Conduct Committee* are somewhat different (Table 4). The most frequent are:

- personal behaviour – most often abuse of drugs and alcohol by the doctor;
- abuse of professional privileges – prescribing of dangerous drugs and false certification;
- abuse of doctor–patient relations – sexual and emotional;
- neglect of responsibilities to patients;
- advertising and canvassing.

The *final outcomes* show that less than one-third of RMPs were erased or suspended with different rates in the various groups.

Table 4   GMC: Professional Conduct Committee

Types of case	Percentage of total	Percentage erased or suspended from Medical Register in each type
Personal behaviour	56	29
Abuse of personal privileges	20	43
Abuse of doctor–patient relations	14	31
Neglect of personal responsibilities to patients	8	19
Advertising/canvassing	2	20
All	—	31

Source: *Annual Reports of GMC*, 1973–1983

Family Practitioner Committees (FPC)

The FPCs are responsible for general practitioners, dental and ophthalmic services. Complaints against these practitioners are assessed by the staff and deputed members of FPC. If the matter is of possible serious significance then it is referred to the Medical Service Committee (for GPs).

The numbers of cases referred to these committees in England, and those in which a breach of regulations was found, from 1977 to 1982 (Table 5 and Figure 3) were 720 per year or 3 per cent of all GP principals. A breach was found in 17 per cent. For general dental practitioners a breach was found in 47 per cent, but the criteria were very different in the two groups.

Table 5   FPCs: mean annual numbers referred to Medical Services Committee and percentages in which breach was found (1977–1982)

	General practitioners	General dental practitioners
Mean annual numbers referred to Medical Service Committees	720	290
Percentage in which breach of regulations was found	17%	47%

Source: *Health and Personal Social Service Statistics*, 1982, Table 5.4

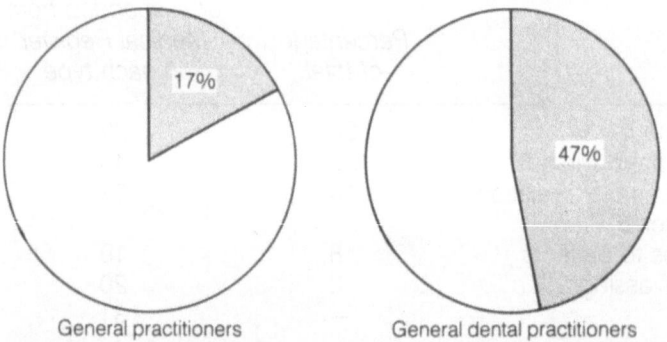

General practitioners   General dental practitioners

Figure 3   Medical Service Committees: percentages in which breach was found (1977–1982) (Health and Personal Social Service Statistics, *1982, Table 5.14*)

Klein (*Complaints against doctors:* London: Charles Knight, 1973) reviewed the data for 1949–1971 and found that the causes of all *complaints* (not only those of Medical Service Committees) were: (see Figure 4):

● bad manners by GP and staff   35 per cent
● failure to visit at home   14 per cent
● failure of appointment system or inability to
   contact GP   14 per cent
● inadequate examination and treatment   16 per cent
● others   22 per cent

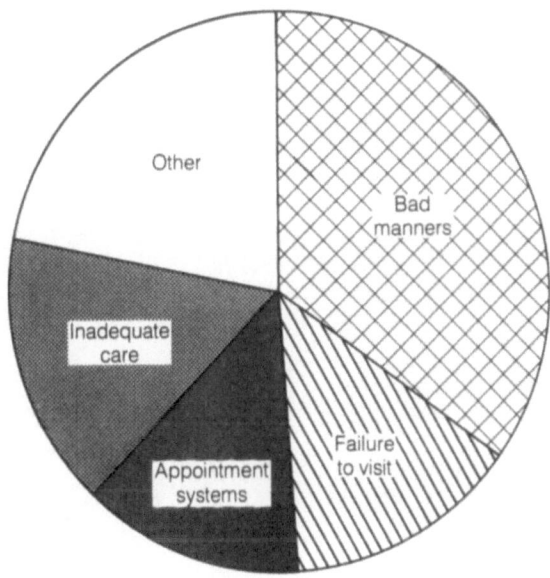

Figure 4 Causes of all FPC complaints

Of those referred to the *Medical Service Committees* the most frequent reasons were:

- failure to visit at home;
- inadequate treatment.

Hospital and community services

Of all complaints received by district and regional health authorities in England in 1981, 40.6 per cent (6603) were about clinical judgements by doctors (Figure 5). This is a rate of 1.5 per 1000 discharges from hospital:

- other complaints   9671 (59.4%)
- about clinical judgement   6603 (40.6%)

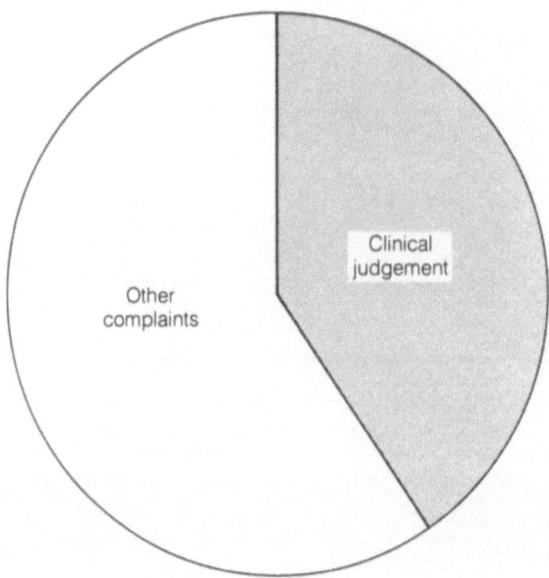

Figure 5   Complaints against hospital doctors (clinical judgement) 1981, as percentage of all hospital complaints

---

COMMENT

- The selected data quoted represent serious cases that must be the tip of an iceberg of dissatisfaction. Nevertheless, it is important to separate the more serious cases in which serious professional misconduct was found proven by GMC or breach of regulations by MSC from the grumbles and annoyances that relate more to personal factors than to failures of the NHS system.
- It is estimated that there are 8323 *complaints about doctors* in a year (some will be sent to more than one body).
- *General Medical Council* annually receives 1000 complaints but only 2.6 per cent of these reach the Professional Conduct Committee for public hearing.

256   COMPLAINTS

- *Family Practitioner Committees*: 720 annual complaints; a breach of regulations was found in 17 per cent.
- *Hospital services*: 6603 complaints about clinical care, a rate of 1.5 per 1000 deaths and discharges from hospital. In very few is any neglect found.

CHAPTER 18

COSTS

The NHS is one of the top employers and spenders. Employing over 1 million workers its proportion of the gross national product (GNP) is around 6 per cent.

TOTAL NHS EXPENDITURE, CRUDE AND INFLATION-ADJUSTED

The *crude annual expenditure* of the NHS (not adjusted for inflation) is rising each year, reaching over £15,000 million in 1983 (Figure 1). When the *costs are adjusted for inflation* (Figure 2) and

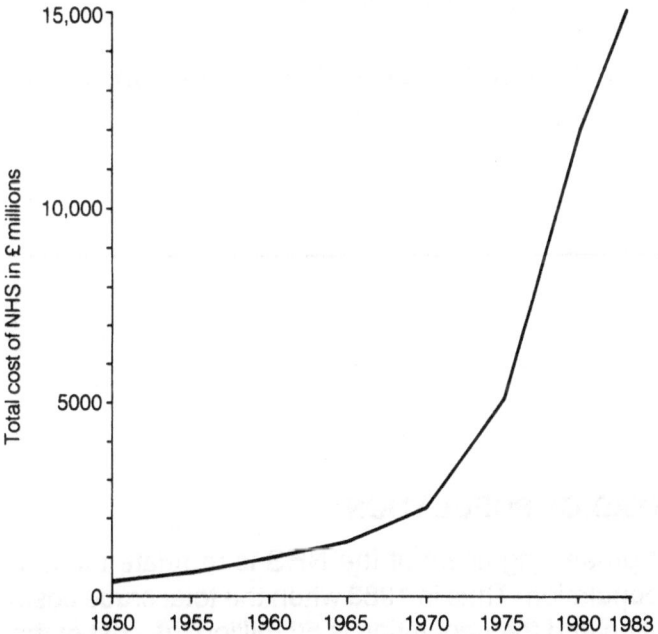

Figure 1   Total costs of NHS, 1949–1983 (not adjusted for inflation) (From Office of Health Economics (OHE), Compendium of Health Statistics, *1981, Table 1.1)*

presented at 1949 constant prices the increase has been almost 4-fold, from £437 million in 1949 to £1500 million (estimated) in 1983.

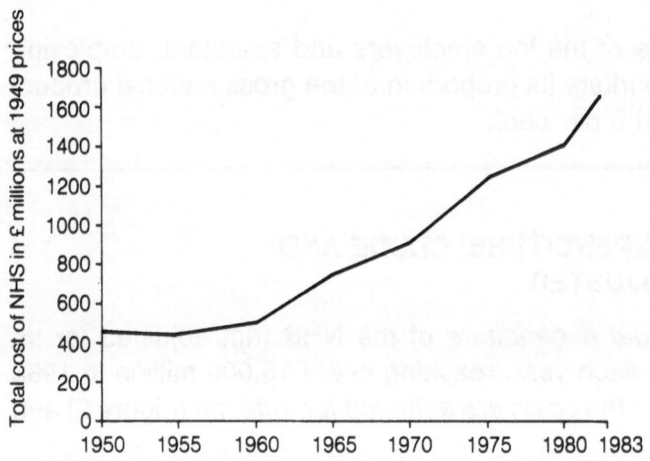

Figure 2   Total costs of NHS, 1949–1983 (at 1949 prices and adjusted for inflation) (OHE Compendium, 1981, Table 1.1)

COSTS PER HEAD OF POPULATION

Another way of presenting costs of the NHS is to relate them to persons in the population. Thus in 1983 when the total crude costs are £15,000 million and the population is 56 million the cost of the NHS per person is £268 in that year – a remarkable increase from the £9 in 1949 (Figure 3). The estimated annual cost in 1983 for each person aged over 75 is £765 and for 65–74 is £310.

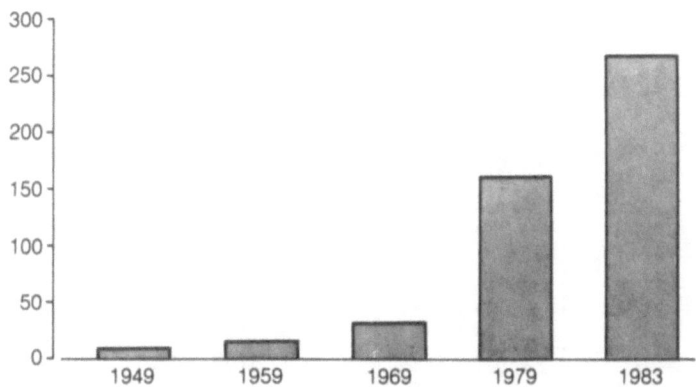

Figure 3 Total annual NHS expenditure per head of population 1949–1983 (unadjusted for inflation) (OHE Compendium, *1981*, Table 1.1)

INTERNATIONAL COMPARISONS

Compared with other countries the NHS is cheap both in costs per capita and as percentage of GNP for 1979 (Figures 4 and 5).

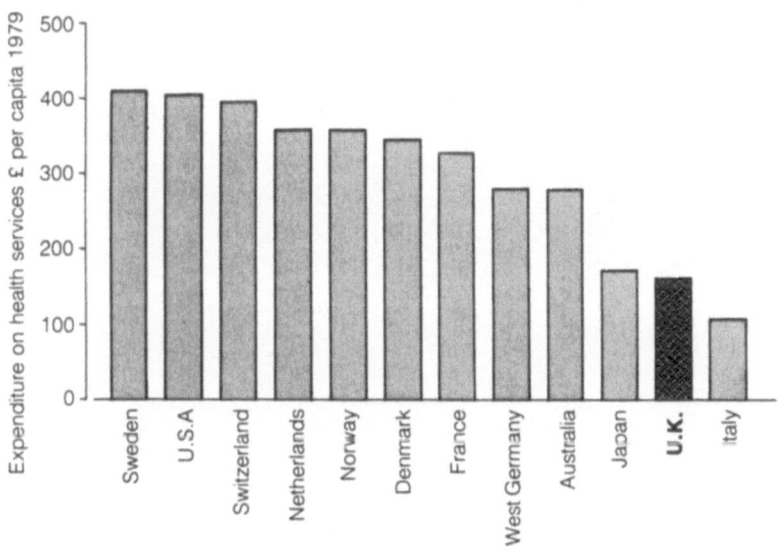

Figure 4 Per capita expenditure on health in 1979 in various countries (OHE Compendium, *1981*, Table 1.2)

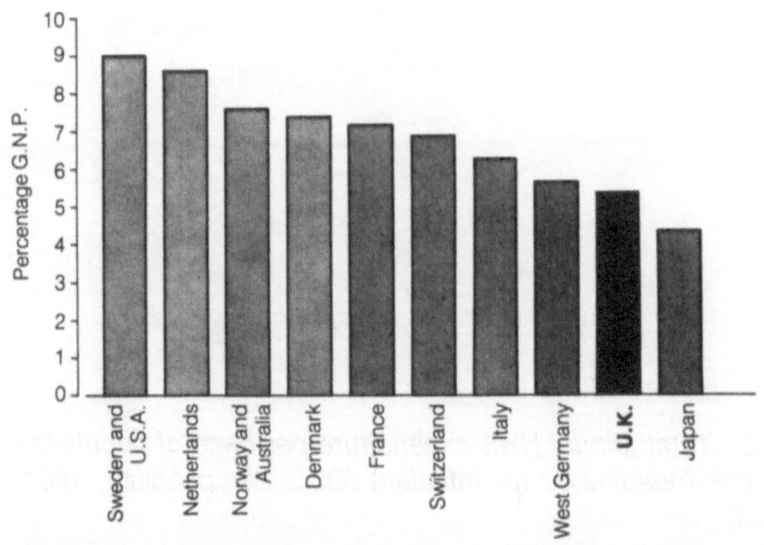

Figure 5   Health expenditure as percentages of GNP in 1979 in various countries (OHE Compendium, *1981, Table 1.2*)

WHERE THE MONEY COMES FROM

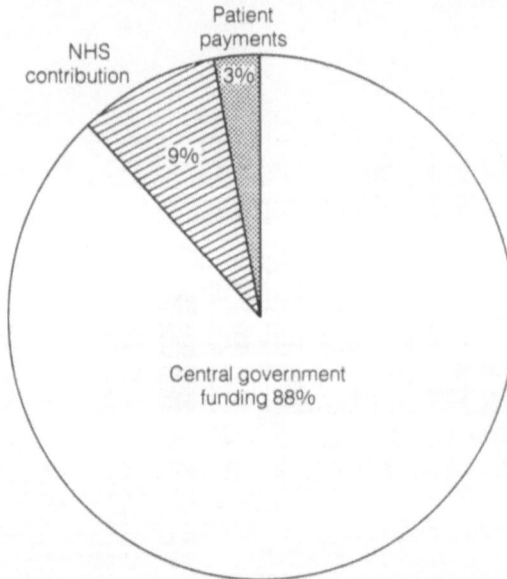

Figure 6   NHS – Sources of finance (1980) (OHE Compendium, *1981, Table 1.5*)

262   COSTS

Almost all funding of the NHS comes from central government Exchequer contributions; that is from taxation and other sources. Less than 10 per cent derives from NHS payments by patients for prescription charges and for other payments (Figure 6).

WHERE THE MONEY GOES

Hospitals

The hospital services are the most expensive part of the NHS (Figure 7) and their share of the total costs has increased, whilst that of the general medical services has decreased (Figure 8). The proportion spent on drugs has remained unchanged at 10 per cent from 1950 to 1980.

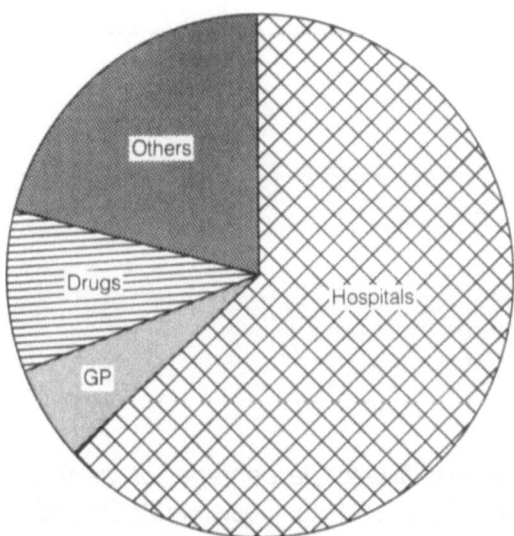

*Figure 7   NHS gross expenditure – share on hospitals, general practice and drugs (1980) (*OHE Compendium, *Table 1.3)*

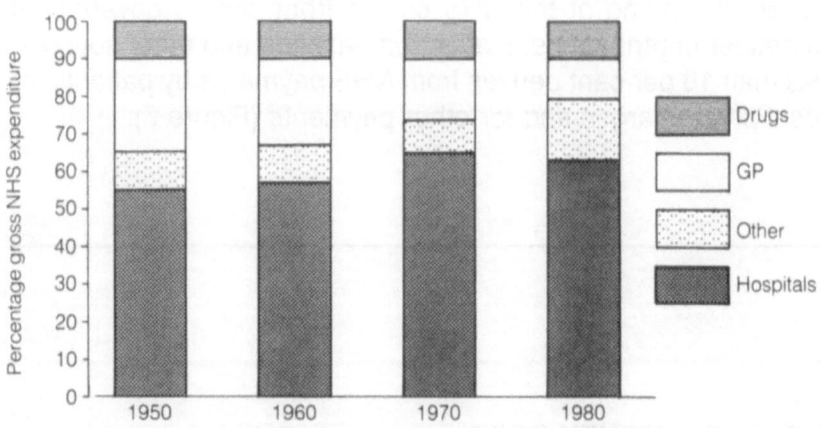

Figure 8   Percentages of NHS gross expenditure spent on hospitals and general practice

Within the hospital costs two-thirds are staff salaries and 23 per cent are for supplies and equipment (Figure 9).

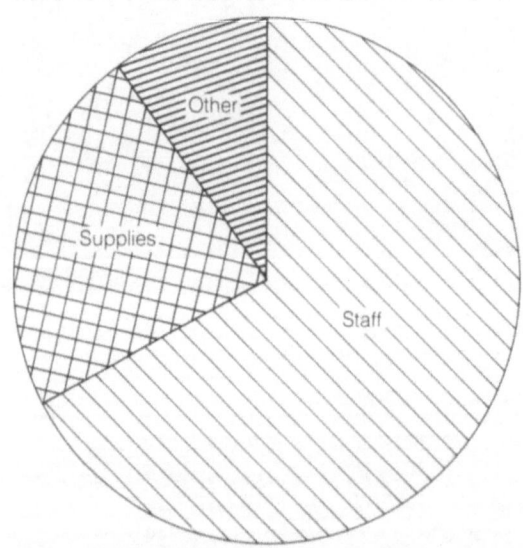

Figure 9   NHS hospital expenditure: percentage of services (1981–1982) (DHSS: Health Care and its Costs; HMSO, 1983, Figure 1)

HOSPITAL COSTS FOR SPECIFIC SERVICES

The *hospital inpatient costs* per day in different units are shown in Figure 10, with maternity departments as the most expensive of the general departments.

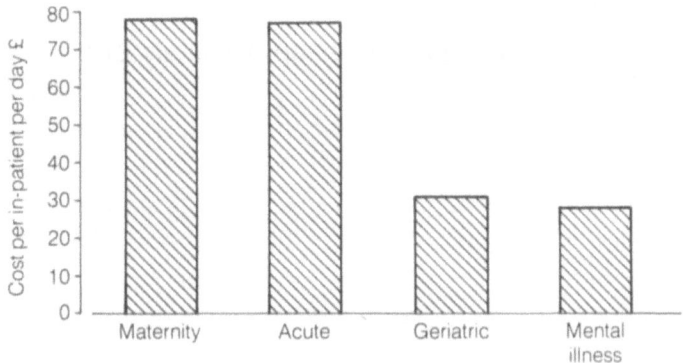

Figure 10   Hospital inpatient costs per day of various units (DHSS: Health Care and its Costs; HMSO, 1983, Figure 3)

Statistics on the average *costs of some hospital services* (Table 1) provide an awareness of their respective levels.

Table 1   Average net costs to NHS of each attendance outpatient and accident–emergency departments, and for each inpatient day

	1978/1979 (£)	1983 (estimated) (£)
Outpatient	10	15
Accident–emergency	6	7.50
Inpatient, per day	37	45

Source: *OHE Compendium*, 1981, Tables 1.11 and 1.12

FAMILY PRACTITIONER SERVICES

Family practitioner services (FPS) comprise general practitioners, pharmacists, dentists and opticians.

The FPS share of the NHS gross expenditure fell from 35 per cent in 1950 to 22 per cent in 1980 (Figure 11). Within the FPS the distribution of expenditure among the four sectors for which the Family Practitioner Committees are responsible shows that the cost of pharmaceuticals prescribed by general practitioners was 46 per cent (Figure 12).

A consultation plus prescription costs approximately £10.

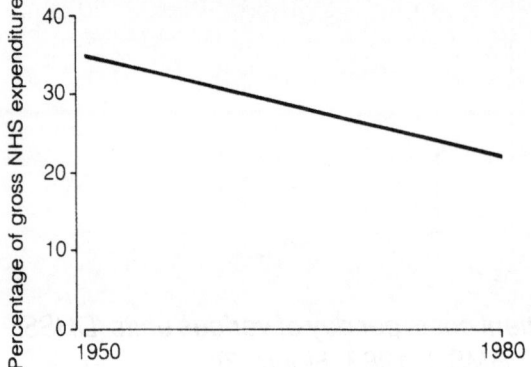

Figure 11 Family practitioner services' share of gross NHS expenditure 1950–1980 (OHE Compendium, 1981, Table 1.3)

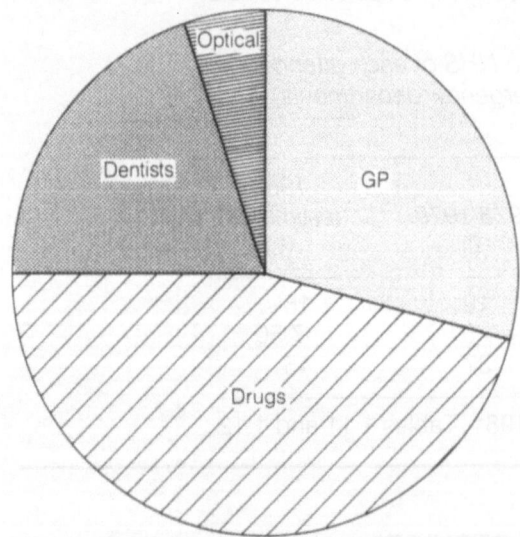

Figure 12 Proportionate costs of family practitioner services (DHSS, Health Care and its Costs; HMSO, 1983, Figure 1)

COMMENTS

- The NHS accounts for 6 per cent of *GNP*.
- *Cost* in 1983 is over £15,000 million.
- Cost at *constant 1949 prices* has quadrupled.
- Cost is £268 *per person* in UK.
- These costs are less than in many *other developed countries*; the amount of money spent on health services is directly related to the affluence of a nation – the higher the GNP the greater proportion of it will be spent on health.
- *Sources of funds* for NHS:
  - 88 per cent from central government (from indirect taxation);
  - 9 per cent from National Insurance contributions;
  - 3 per cent from direct payments by patients, i.e. prescription charges, etc.
- *Where the money goes:*
  - hospital service   63 per cent
  - general practice   6 per cent
  - drugs   10 per cent
  - other   21 per cent
- *Hospital costs:*
  - staff   67 per cent
  - supplies   23 per cent
  - other   10 per cent
- *Hospital item costs* (1983):
  - inpatient, per day   £45
  - outpatient attendance   £15
  - accident–emergency attendance   £7.50
- A GP consultation and prescription costs £10.
- The costings, allocations and cost-benefits are *crude and insufficient* for a service employing over 1 million and costing £15,000 million in 1983.

INDEX

abortions 64–6
accidents
  and alcohol consumption 51–4
  in the home 54–5
  road traffic 53–4
accommodation, local authority 59–60
acute wheezy chests/asthma 216–17
alcohol 51–3
allocated beds 94–5
anaesthetic deaths 224–30
anaesthetists 227–9

babies 182
birth rate 4, 6, 179
birth weight and class 79–80
blindness 56–7

cancers 219–22
car, use of 29
careers 127
causes of death 6–7, 38–9, 41
cervical cytology 197–201
cervical screening 82
chemists and drug stores 98, 161–2
child minders and nurseries 61
children 3
  in care 61–3
cirrhosis of the liver 51–2
community dental services 188–91
community homes 98–101
community ophthalmic
    services 185–6
complaints against doctors 249–57
consultants 110–12
  distribution 35
contraception 204–7
costs
  family practitioner services 265–6
  hospital services 263–5
  NHS, per head 260–1
  NHS, total 259
  prescribing 156–8
crime 70

deafness 57
death rates 4, 5, 6
  and social class 74–9
deaths 4
  infants 84–5
  maternal 84
  see also mortality
dental services 81–2
dentists 188–9
diabetes 213–14
dialysis and transplantation 231–47
disabled 55–6
dispensing doctors 161
district, NHS 35
divorce 66–8
domiciliary consultations 137–8
domiciliary midwives 184
drug use 49–50

education 30–2
  employment 21
elderly people 4
employment 16–21
  and education 21, 23
  by industry 17
  by sector 17–18
epilepsy 218–19

family planning 204–7
family practitioner committees (FFC)
    253–5
general dental practitioners 117
General Medical Council (GMC)
    250–3
general practice 132–47
  annual persons consulting 45–7,
    133–4
  domicilary consultations 137
  grades of disease 144–7
  and medical schools 123–4
  morbidity in 43–5
  referrals to hospital 136
general practice units 96–7

general practitioners 113–16
  distribution 35
  maternity beds 183
  numbers 113
  persons per GP 113
  profiles 114–15
  work profile 134–5
gross weekly earnings 13

haemodialysis 236
handicapped 55–6
  hostels and homes for 101
health service 80–2
high blood pressure 210–13
holiday entitlement 21, 24
home help services 58–9
hospital and community services,
    complaints against 255–6
hospitals 91–5
  admissions per consultant 149–50
  allocated and occupied beds 94–5
  bed size 92
  inpatients 147–50
  medical staff 108–12
  non-psychiatric and psychiatric 93
  numbers 91
  outpatients, morbidity in 43
  services 139–41
hostels and homes for mentally ill and
    handicapped 101
house ownership 27
housing 27–9

illegitimate births 69
immigration 9
immunization 81, 201–3
income 13–6
infant deaths 179–80
inpatients, psychiatric 164

late antenatal bookings 80
leisure 32
levels of administration 88–9
levels of care 87–9
life expectancy 8
live births 4
local authority
  homes 98–101
  services 15
  social services 117–18
low birthweights 182

marriage
maternal deaths 84
maternal mortality 181
maternal and perinatal mortality
    203–4
maternity services 179–84
meals service 58
medical schools and general practice
    123–7
medical staff, increases 82–3
medical students 121–3
medical training, cost of 124
medication 131–2
mental handicap 172–6
mentally ill, hostels and homes for
    101
migration 9
morbidity 35–48
mortality 35–48, 85
  by occupation 77–9
  regional variations in 79

newspapers 32–3
NHS
  expenditure 259–67
  finance 262–3
  personnel 105 ff.
  structure and roles 87 ff.

occupational class 85
occupied beds 94–5
OTC drugs 156
outpatients 150–1
  morbidity in 43
  psychiatric 167–8

pathology and radiology requests
    139
pay beds 102
peptic ulcers 215–16
peritoneal dialysis 236–41
personnel 105–19
place of death 36–7
population, UK 1 ff.
  age-sex distribution 2
  children 3
  dependent 5
  elderly 4
  working 16
population, world 10
postgraduate examination pass rates
    126–7

pregnancy, termination 208-10
prescribing 155-62
  costs 156-8
  drugs 156-7, 160
  exemptions from charges 160
  numbers 159
prevention 197
private medical services 102-3
private and voluntary homes 100-3
psychiatric hospitals 93-5
  admissions 166
  deaths and discharges 165
  diagnosis 168-9
  hospital resources 163-4
  inpatients 164
  lengths of stay 170-2
  outpatients 167-8
psychiatry 163-76

real household disposable income 13
rheumatoid arthritis 217-18

school-leavers 32
school medical service 193-6
self care 130-1, 142-3
self check 210
self-medication 131-2, 156
senior house officer (SHO) posts 125
sexually transmitted diseases 63-4
sight tests 186-8
smears 199-201

smoking 49-50
SMR *see* standardized mortality ratio
social class 73-85
social services 117
specialties 110-11
staff, NHS 106-8
standardized mortality ratios 39, 40
  high blood pressure 210-13
suicides 69-70
surgical operations 42-3

taxes 15-16
telephones 29
termination of pregnancy 208-10;
  see also abortion
thyroid disorders 215
time spent at work 21
transplantation 231-47

UK population 1-11
unemployment 16-22
usage of health service, by social class
  80-2
utilization of health care 129

vocational training for general practice
  125-6

weekly earnings 14
whooping cough 202-3
working population 16